i

YOU TOO CAN 'DO' HEALTH!

By

OLIVE HICKMOTT

&

SARAH KNIGHTON

The names, characters and incidents portrayed in this book are the work of the authors' imagination. Any resemblance to actual persons, living or dead, events or localities, is entirely coincidental.

ISBN 978-1-904312-30-7

First published in 2007

© Copyright 2007 Olive Hickmott & Sarah Knighton

Although every effort has been made to assure the accuracy of the information contained in this book as of the date of publication, nothing herein should be construed as giving specific treatment advice. In addition, the application of the techniques to specific circumstances can present complex issues that are beyond the scope of this book. This publication is intended to provide general information pertaining to developing these skills.

Published in the UK by MX Publishing Ltd, 10 Kingfisher Close, Stanstead Abbotts, Hertfordshire, SG12 8LQ. www.mxpublishing.co.uk

Cover design and graphics by Sarah Fawkes: www.sarahfawkesdesign.co.uk

You too can 'do' health

This is a story for everyone.

One person's journey of self-development and self-awareness to health and well-being.

Using the tools of NLP, universal energy and the secret law of attraction, learn how to map your own journey and achieve the health you want.

Visit the web site:

www.youtoocandohealth.com

Dedication

To my husband for always believing in my health; my family for never allowing me to wallow in self-pity and everyone else I have met; who have knowingly or not, been an influence on my journey … Sarah Knighton

For my family and friends, to whom I am eternally grateful for their support and patience; may you stay blessed with good health – I love you all … Olive Hickmott

About the authors

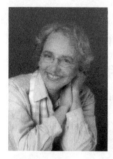 **Olive Hickmott** is an NLP Master Practitioner, Energetic NLP Practitioner and certified coach working with individuals and corporations to enable personal growth in many aspects of their lives. In corporate life, which she left in 1990, she was an engineering director. She founded her own business, Empowering Health, and is director of the Hickmott Partnership. Her passion is enabling people to achieve their goals in any aspect of their lives, especially their health, often helping people with acute and chronic illness return to health. She says "it is just a privilege to see what individuals can achieve, when they realise how their mind, body and spirit are all interlinked; so they can decide just how they want to be."

Sarah Knighton is a certified coach as well as being an NLP Master 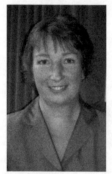 Practitioner, with an additional certification in health and an Energetic NLP Practitioner. Sarah has been interested in health and healing from the age of 4, when she nursed all her toys back to health from various malaises! Sarah ran her own part-time complementary therapies practice whilst running a full time training consultancy within the financial sector of the City. Having given up the training consultancy to concentrate on Health Coaching, she now works with many different health issues that people come to her with; however, her specialities are working with those affected and affected by breast cancer and those who have reading and spelling challenges.

Acknowledgements

There are many people we wish to thank for their help and influence in writing this book. In particular:

Our wonderful teachers, who include; Robert Dilts, Tim Hallbom, Ian McDermott, Suzi Smith and Lutz Wesel, for the ideas and thinking that have contributed much to the authors' ability to write this book.

All our trainers and colleagues who have helped us on our own journeys.

Art Giser, founder of EnergeticNLP (www.energeticnlp.com), not only for his assistance to our spiritual growth and healing skills, but the very practical contribution of his work, which he has gifted us for incorporation in two chapters of this book.

The research and work we have done for this book, results from inspiring collaborations between Olive Hickmott and Sarah Knighton. We have relied very much on each other to challenge our thinking and through this process, help so many individuals achieve what they have wanted.

Thanks to the clients who we have worked with for their invaluable contribution to our thinking, for sharing and showing us the beauty of their health and wellness, and allowing us to develop the approach used in this book. We continually learn so much, by understanding their experiences, and giving us the source of new perspectives.

And by no means least, thanks to our families, who not only read parts of the script, but challenged our thinking and above all, supported us throughout the project.

The extracts on page 91 are from Research done by Dr. Ronald Grossarth-Maticek on 3,055 elderly residents in Heidelberg, Germany, published in *The Attitude Factor - Extend Your Life by Changing the Way You Think,* Thomas R Blakeslee (iUniverse.com , 2004); the extract on page 93 is from the film *Bambi,* Walt Disney (originally released in 1942); the extract on page 136 is from *To be honest with you,* Linford Christie (Penguin Books Ltd; New Ed edition, 1996) ; the extract on page 225 is from *Charlie and the Chocolate Factory,* Roald Dahl (Puffin Books; New Ed edition, 2001); Short'nin' bread, mentioned on page 297 can be found at http://kids.niehs.nih.gov/lyrics/shortninbread.htm ;

NEW PERSPECTIVES

With every new day you have a choice; a choice to do things differently.

If you choose the same actions as yesterday, you will get the same results.

Try another way.

Preface

By Olive Hickmott and Sarah Knighton

We have written this book for those interested in investigating the mind-body connection to health and their own self-development.

We are both on our own healing journeys; the catalyst for these journeys was our growth, often driven by our own ill health.

Throughout our own separate journeys we have learnt an enormous amount about ourselves through the complementary practices of Neuro Linguistic Programming (NLP), coaching, energy, nutrition and exercise.

We are now both health coaches and the objective of this book is to enable anyone to realise just what might be possible and enable their learning. Many of our clients have asked us what they can read to accelerate change. Even our colleagues ask us for book recommendations of our work for their clients.

The ideas held within this easy to read story will help everyone to make sense of their own experiences and move them towards their goals. The use of a story enables the reader, to take just what they want, at that time, without pressure.

The journey you take is always very personal. Sarah's was to overcome cancer whilst Olive's has been to work through minor health challenges and survive peritonitis.

The routes you take will inevitably be different at every bend in the road. Just a few of the "golden nuggets" you may take from this work are: learning from your experiences, however severe; taking from them the positive learning; being curious; getting in touch with yourself and firing your growth.

Illness drives you to explore for yourself, no-one else can do it for you. Neither of us would be the Health Coaches we are today, without having been driven to explore through our own illnesses.

When we started this work, health coaching was almost unheard of, now it is gathering more and more acceptability and accessibility, as individuals realise that the techniques have to offer some really simple and practical benefits that are available to everyone.

Olive has often encouraged individuals to think of a metaphor for themselves, asking, "just how do you think of yourself?" Just this one question can have a significant affect on your health.

This is her personal metaphor:

"I think of myself as a tree, growing strong and tall, whilst letting the wind of change blow through the branches and generating new growth. Amongst the branches I can see small animals such as squirrels and birds happily going about their day to day business and co-existing with the insects and mites in harmony. Not only do others experience and are inspired by the outward signs of growth but, underground, away from public view, the roots reach out further and further, deep into the subsoil, to nurture my own growth, stabilising me to support my ability to help others. As we all know, we need to look after ourselves to be in place to look after others – although we often do the opposite by neglecting ourselves and then find we are unable to give others the support we would like to. Our roots need to be strong for us and for them.

Then there is how the seasons affect the tree – the strength in the winter to withstand the elements; the new growth and blossom to show off the inner natural beauty everywhere in the spring; flowering during the summer; in autumn letting go of the leaves so valued such a short time ago but now no longer needed. And at the same time you can celebrate spreading the seeds for another season, to give so many others the same opportunities for their very individual growth."

Question what you read in this book! For example, why do some people always seem to be healthy, where perhaps you are not? This type of self-talk is invaluable for sorting out your own experiences, but remember not to let your self-talk limit what you can achieve.

It will be better if you can clear your mind about any medical diagnosis, prognosis, or 'what might happen next', and put all that to one side whilst you read this book.

Let the words of the book flow past you, you will take just

what you need at this time. The more you become curious about your own situation, the more answers you will get, the more changes you will want to do, the more you will be able to achieve and learn about yourself.

If you require further assistance for yourself or members of your community, you will find our details in the front and back of this book. You only have to ask, we are always delighted to assist.

The information, advice and suggestions published within this book are not a substitute for proper medical consultation for physical, mental and psychological illnesses.
This book is not intended to replace the services of a qualified medical practitioner.
Information in this book is provided as complementary to other avenues you may be pursuing.

PART 1

INSPIRATIONS FOR CHANGE

90% of your thoughts today, are the same as they were yesterday and will be the same tomorrow – unless you make a change.

(R Bandler, J Grinder et al.)

Chapter 1:
The Chemist Sets A Challenge

Harry Winthrop

Harry Winthrop was Mr Normal, 42, with a wife (Jenny), 2 children and a cat, working as a team leader in an advertising agency.

As he sits in the doctor's waiting room, he realises that he has read most of the magazines before and then starts to count up just how many times he has been to see the doctor this year. It must be 7 or 8 and it is only June! He always seems to be going with different problems, none of them life threatening and he is generally given a prescription for some type of medication. On two occasions this year he has been sent for a blood test and when the results have come back, he is assured there is nothing wrong. This really annoys him as he's convinced there is something actually wrong; otherwise why does he keep catching all these bugs, colds and flu, and getting aches and pains all over his body? He just knows there's something more going on in his body and that the doctors are fobbing him off with pills.

On this occasion, he visits the doctor because he is feeling really run down, has no energy and is given another prescription. It is suggested he tries to get a little more fresh air, exercise and improve his diet.

As he leaves the surgery he is thinking to himself. 'This is all very well, but I know all of this and I can't seem to do it, it is just too much effort! The doctor ought to be able to give me some kind of magic pill to solve this'.

Funny how things happen

Whilst waiting in the chemist for his prescription, that he has little faith in working, he finds a card on the counter for Mary Hibbert, which says 'You too can 'do' health!' Harry immediately thinks that someone is either having a laugh or, perhaps, they indeed have found the magic pill!

He asks the pharmacist what he knows about Mary, "Mary is great, and gets some fantastic results, but it won't work for you."

"Why not?" said Harry, already affronted at the tone of voice used by the pharmacist.

"Because you have to *want* to change, possibly change your lifestyle, change some of your habits, change the way you think about things and frankly, I don't see you doing any of that."

"Why not?" snapped Harry, for this was getting somewhat monotonous and Harry was becoming quite annoyed by this time.

"Well, I am sorry if I am offending you, but I have owned this chemist for 5 years and I have filled so many prescriptions for you and I don't think that any of the inconvenience that you have been through with your health has convinced you to change. So, what chance does Mary have! You have to start taking responsibility for your own health."

"But I do." "When I am ill, I go to the doctor and come in here for my prescription to be filled."

"Yes you do do that, but do you always take the medication correctly? It doesn't just jump out of the bottle you know! What about making a few changes that might prevent you being ill so often. That would tell me that at least you are interested in your own health. And then there's all that moaning about the weather, your kids, the length of time you had to wait to see the doctor, in fact about anything and everything. Have you not noticed that people who moan all the time are miserable? Being negative is bound to affect your health in the long run. It is a fact that happy people live longer!"

Warming to his topic, the pharmacist continued.

"I warn you, Mary is great but she won't help you unless you want to change. You will need to be curious about how you can think differently, challenge and shift some of your views on life, for example the one that says your health is everyone else's responsibility but yours!

Mary can only work with people who are open minded, and she will make that very clear. I should also warn you that it seems more difficult for us males to do this than for women. This is, possibly something to do with that expression about men being an island. Often we just resist help, thinking we have to do everything ourselves, but most of us wouldn't have passed our driving test without a teacher – so where is the logic in that?!

If you are open minded and curious, you will learn lots about how you can affect your health, getting enormous insights from within yourself about the changes you can make and it is FUN! You will learn much you didn't know, you didn't know about yourself and generally about how we humans work."

Harry was getting fed up with this lecture on how wonderful this Mary woman was. How did the pharmacist know so much anyway? Harry decided to ask him.

"It is all very well you telling me all this, but how do I know, that you know, what you are talking about? You could be married to her for all I know and just saying all this to get business."

The pharmacist burst out laughing!

"Oh dear, you *are* a sceptical one. No, I am certainly not married to Mary! I know 'so much' as you refer to it, because I have done some work with her myself in the past; quite a lot of work in fact. I still go and see her every now and then, when I want a bit of help unsticking something that I can't quite work through on my own.

Let me just tell you why I originally went to see Mary.

"Several years ago I had cancer, I underwent months of medical treatment and it was great that they got rid of the cancer but it left me feeling as if the fire brigade had been in. The fire was out but my house was left a smouldering wreck which I needed to start rebuilding, and rebuilding it in such a way that the cancer would not return."

That took the wind out of Harry's sails! He calmed down a bit as he stood looking at the pharmacist, but still felt aggrieved that the pharmacist had dismissed the idea that he would see Mary.

"OK then, what else do you think you know about me?"

"Honestly?"

Harry nodded

"At the moment I think you are probably quite 'stuck' in a negative sort of way. Things seem to happen to you and you have become a victim of them. You let life and the events in it run you, rather than being proactive about your life.

However, it is up to you to take the first step. You really don't need to live like this. I have seen all sorts of people, who have worked with Mary, have achieved amazing results to dramatically improve their health. The question is, do you want to make a difference to your health and your life?"

Harry picked up his filled prescription, turned to leave and as he walked towards the door, a voice inside his head said 'well what have you got to lose?' He went back and picked up a card from the counter, checked for a phone number, looked at the pharmacist, "I bet I can do this," and left.

The pharmacist chuckled to himself, 'Just the sort of motivation he needed, he might just give it a good go now to prove me wrong'

Harry makes an appointment

When he got home, before he had even taken his coat off or let anyone talk him out of it, Harry phoned Mary Hibbert. He immediately realised she was a very straight talking woman, who said exactly what she thought.

She explained that the results he achieved, would be down to his own efforts and the amount of curiosity he showed. She booked him in for his first session the following week and suggested he might like to book another 3 sessions when he came, so that he could get some momentum going.

"Do you mean I might be fixed in just 4 sessions?" he asked Mary, somewhat amazed.

"That is up to you. Think of what you are doing as being a journey. You started your journey of exploration when the chemist challenged your thinking. That's when you decided to go and explore.

When we meet, you will get many more insights about the changes you can make to achieve the health you want. It is completely up to you how you implement and integrate these into your life. You may find that you get the results you want very quickly. Or, what you are starting may become a lifelong journey of self-understanding and self-development."

"You mean I have to see you for the rest of my life?"

"Oh heavens, no" laughed Mary. "I'll be like a guide book you might want to dip into as you explore new places. Think of your first session as the plane tickets for your journey. During your sessions, you may well find a lot of things change and you will be a lot clearer about what steps you want to take next."

Having made his appointment, Harry spent the rest of the day intrigued and very curious about what he could change and how it would change his health.

His conversation with Mary had set him thinking. His mind was racing and not with the same thoughts he normally had. When he went to bed that night he had several unusual dreams.

Chapter 2:
Harry Starts His Journey

By the time the tyres of his car crept over the crisp gravel, Harry was full of questions. How would he know whether he could do this, or would it be just something else he would fail at; just like the pharmacist said.

He really didn't know what to expect, so here he was, ringing the front door bell. He had no idea what was inside and part of him didn't even want to know. Would it be scary? Would he have to address questions he had done a great job of hiding under the carpet all these years? Was it going to be hard work? And how an earth was this going to be FUN?

As he waited by the door Harry had a strange feeling in his stomach, like being on a roller coaster, one moment he was elated that he was taking some new steps to improve his health and that this opportunity offered what he really wanted, whilst a moment later he could be dropping into panic – this might be change with a capital C and he didn't really like change.

A lady opened the door with a big smile, "Hello, you must be Harry, I am Mary Hibbert, do come in."

Harry had imagined Mary looking very severe and strict for some reason, a bit like one of his old school teachers, who had always been telling him to do better; but she wasn't a bit like them. She seemed to have a sense of calm that enveloped her and everything around her. She looked younger than he had imagined too. He vaguely wondered how old she was, but it was too difficult to tell and he wasn't about to ask her!

It's a two-way street

Mary welcomed him in and they settled into a lovely airy room with comfortable chairs.

"Before we start any work, I'd like to get a small amount of paperwork out of the way if you don't mind.

This is the agreement my clients and I work to. I'd like you to read it and then sign your acceptance to the statements that are written for both our benefits. If there's anything you are not sure about, please do ask me and I'll elaborate for you."

She handed Harry the agreement, which he read and
signed, handing the completed form back to Mary, she
thanked him and put it to one side. (see appendix 1)

The gift of time

Mary made him feel very comfortable. She said that in
this first session she would be explaining a little more
about the processes they would be going through, and
giving him the gift of time:

> Time to think for himself.
> Time to consider what he really wanted.
> Time to learn something about himself.
> Time to appreciate his strengths and resources.
> Time to explore how he saw the world.
> Time to explain what he felt about his health; the stuff
> he knew but thought it sounded silly to say.
> Time to start being curious and getting insights.
> Time to understand intent.
> Time to put my past to one side.

In this session Mary would be explaining a few things
about 'how things work around here' so that he had a
context for their ongoing work.

Firstly she introduced herself, her background and training and whilst she wasn't medically trained, she respected the role that medics played, as an invaluable part of our society.

She then went on to describe how she came to be a health coach and why she was so committed to the work she did. How working with a coach helps you move forward from where you are now, towards where you want to be. How health coaching assists people get more in touch with themselves and what this understanding means for them.

Mary explained that her role was to guide his exploration, help him listen to his own wisdom better and give him the tools to change. He was the one that would be doing all the work!

'That must be what the chemist meant when he said he didn't think I would be able to do it; because I was so used to just taking a pill for the latest symptom' Harry thought to himself.

Mary then explained to Harry how a state of dis-ease or illness is where our body is out of balance; the key is to determine how we could bring it back to balance, health and well-being. It wasn't about offering a quick fix – and was certainly quite different from the medical model, although completely complementary to it.

What she did hope and wish for, was for each person she worked with, to incorporate into their own health programme what they found out about themselves, during each session.

"It's like getting your best friend to help you on a 24-7 basis."

The way things work around here

Mary explained that it was no accident that they were sitting in the Entrance Hall. This was where everyone's story began. The Entrance Hall is where you greet people, make them feel comfortable and give them an idea of how the rest of the house is organised. She explained that metaphorically, Harry would be exploring his own 'Manor House' in just the way he wanted to, although she did have some tips for newcomers.

Mary handed him a notebook on the cover it said

'You too can 'do' health'

Even after all that Mary had explained in her introduction, the words '*You too can 'do' health'* emblazoned on the notebook really shocked him. 'Can *I* really 'do' health?', he wondered.

All he had to go on were isolated stories he had heard of people who had achieved great improvements in their health. At the moment, he wasn't even sure what constituted a 'great improvement'.

Now he thought about it, he had heard stories about people who had recovered from operations really quickly, or about the chap that had got over a broken leg in less than the 'normal' healing time. There was even that friend of his aunt's who had got over cancer, but everyone in the family just thought she must have been misdiagnosed.

He could recall several other examples when he thought about it and as he went off on a whole train of thought, he noticed that he had stopped listening. In fact Mary had stopped talking. She had noticed he had drifted off too and had paused.

Once Harry's attention was back, Mary went on to explain that drifting off was quite natural, because he was connecting memories together that had previously been isolated events. Whenever he wanted to follow a useful train of thought he should, and just let her know where his thoughts were taking him.

Gosh thought Harry, this was a surprise. Normally people told him to pay attention; he certainly was being given time to listen to himself.

The notebook was empty, except for some additional information that had been stuck in at the back, which included his agreement with Mary. The information contained background about Health Coaching and Mary's profile. The rest of the notebook was blank sheets of paper.

"Your notebook is for any jottings you want to make about what you learn; the insights you achieve; the things you hope to change and the things that are really important to you. You can write in any way you like as it is now your book."

Mary invited Harry to remain where he was for the moment, think about why he was there, what he wanted to achieve, what achieving would be like and what information he already knew. Harry could take as long as he needed, for this was an invaluable time for both he and Mary to understand his map of the world.

Like most people, Harry knew exactly what he *didn't* want but not what he *did* want.

He didn't want to be this overweight. He didn't want to stay in his current job. He didn't want the kids to shout so loudly all the time. He didn't want to constantly be suffering from this or that and he didn't want to feel so run down all the time.

The first thing Mary did was explain why he should change all these negatives into positives.

"Whenever you say anything, your unconscious listens to you. So, if you say or hear things like 'I don't want to be fat'; because your unconscious cannot understand the word 'don't', it deletes it from what you've said or listened to and hears 'I want to be fat'. Our mind always tries to be right, so it will work away in the background trying to help you be fat, because that is what it thinks you want."

Harry was staggered. All this time he had been thinking of things he didn't want, and his mind was trying it's hardest to give them to him! No wonder he never got anywhere!

"Let's take your first comment about being fat. How could you change that, so that it says what you really want, without any negatives?"

Harry sat quietly pondering on how he could change the sentence. He was so used to using negatives that at first he found it hard and kept coming up with alternatives that still contained negatives, but eventually he began to find words to use instead. They didn't make much sense at first, but with perseverance and Mary's encouragement, he finally ended up with… "I want to be 13 stone and have toned muscles."

He knew he wasn't, but just saying this in a different way, he felt thinner already!

He sat back to think about just what he did want, and
jotting down the headings in his new notebook, explained
to Mary:

"Well, obviously I'd like to change everything I said
earlier, but specifically….

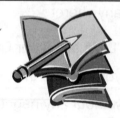

> ⇒ I want to be healthy – I want to run
>   around with the children without
>   being out of breath
> ⇒ I want to understand why I keep
>   getting minor ailments and put a
>   stop to them.
> ⇒ I want to be happy.
> ⇒ I want to stop relying on all of
>   those pills and potions.
> ⇒ Oh, and I'd like to give up
>   smoking too!"

Mary explained "Some of those goals are things you want
to do, whilst others are things you want to run away from.
Using the process we went through just now, could you
rerun those thoughts and feelings and express them as
how you would like to actually *be*. Use the present tense
and get a real sense of what it would be like to be living
that life."

Harry reviewed his list and came up with:

⇒ I am healthy.
⇒ I am happy.
⇒ I am self-healing.
⇒ I am a non-smoker.
⇒ I learn more about myself every
    day."

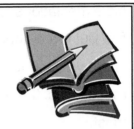

Harry looking bemused thought, 'this was ridiculous, you couldn't change these things so easily'.

"Don't worry Harry, I know you are feeling this is ridiculously easy at this stage, it may well take a bit longer than just a few minutes, but I want you to start to get focused on what you want rather than what you don't want. There is a saying that goes 'whether you think you can or whether you think you can't, you will be right!' I am hoping you can leave what you don't want or think you can't do outside the front door. This is the way to move forward."

He was only minutes into the first session and already light bulbs were coming on in his mind. What would the rest of the session spark off?

Mary explained that in the first session she wanted to set his expectations; or rather, unset them and enable her to find out more about Harry. Further sessions would focus entirely on the topics that were uppermost on his priority list. That is, the ones that he believed would help him most.

"The agenda is always with you, so it is well worth preparing for subsequent sessions."

That sentence also surprised Harry, he had thought subsequent sessions would be focused on what he had done or not done from the previous session. This had been one of the things he had most dreaded – he knew he did too much of this already, what a relief!

Mary explained that it was up to him to decide how to monitor his own progress, she said that it normally worked best to focus on what had gone well and if he was making real progress, his priorities for the next week may have moved on so much, that close monitoring was inappropriate.

He was starting to feel optimistic just hearing this sort of explanation.

Mary carried on to say very clearly, that the work they would do is not a replacement for the years of medical practice or complementary medicine available; what they were doing was complementary to either or both. She would not make any suggestions about changes in medication etc. That was a matter between Harry and his doctor. Health Coaching just offered everyone, using the resources they already possess, the option to focus those resources into positively affecting their health.

Exploring the Mansion

Mary gave Harry a brief description of what he might find in some of the rooms, but stressed that they would be his rooms, and show him how he had constructed his world, or where he could change his current perceptions. It was always different for everyone.

To get him started, she mentioned that he might encounter the following rooms:

> **The Library** – This was where most people started. "It's where you'll find all your past and future events."

The Lake House – "This is a wonderful summer house, set right next to the lake in the grounds of the mansion. This is where you'll learn to let go of the 'baggage' that you are still carrying around and no longer need; the stuff that is 'past its sell-by date' as well as all those large and small traumas that you would rather forget."

This sounded like a great idea to Harry. His wife was always telling him he carried around too much baggage, but never told him how to let go of it – he wondered how he would get rid of it.

The Study – "In this room you'll explore what you think you know and where you think you need to understand more. You might come across a few blank areas in this room. Don't worry about them, they're just space for getting to know what you don't know, you don't know. "

Mary finished her explanation and paused. Then she said "The most important thing is for you to select how and where to start your exploration. Go with what looks, or sounds, or feels right for you. Never mind about what anyone else might think. Oh, and if you come across certain things you identify as values of yours, don't compromise them! From now on, all the decisions are up to you!"

Specifically for Health

Mary asked Harry if he was internally questioning what he had heard and/or thought during the session so far.

"Well yes, some of it anyway."

"Excellent." Mary went on to explain "This self-talk is invaluable for sorting out your experiences, but if all the self-talk gets out of control, the questions you are asking are not going to help you move forward. I am guessing 90% of them are the same as yesterday's and will be the same as tomorrow's, unless you can take another perspective.

It is much better if you can clear your mind about any medical diagnosis or prognosis, or 'what might happen next' thought, and put them to one side for the moment, otherwise, they might limit what you can achieve.

With disease; which I like to pronounce dis-ease because it is what the body is experiencing; the aim is to understand what is going on, so you can have a choice about what you do to get *you* back in control and rebalance your body back to within its 'normal' range.

The scariest thing about dis-ease or illness is feeling you are no longer in control of *you* and things are happening to you quite outside your control.

So the pillars of what we will explore together are:

Making changes and noting what happens.

Helping you to be more in touch with *you* and understand what your body is trying to signal to your mind.

Understanding how your body and mind work together - this will lead you to insights into what is happening to and for you.

Helping you move from being out of balance, back into balance.

Helping you move forward to do the things that are really important to you. (Doing this will help some of the stuff you are currently battling with, fade away and will give you more energy).

Helping you obtain some new perspectives."

As Harry listened to Mary, it sounded like there was a huge mountain to climb. How would they, or more correctly he, achieve anything?

Just as he was thinking this, Mary continued. "My role is to find the best tools for you to use, that will help you move forward and encourage your curiosity and self-discovery.

It may help you to understand a little about your dis-ease, but too much information just gets you more stuck in it and you *become* your dis-ease or illness.

What you really need to find out, is what is happening in you to cause this dis-ease what is out of balance?

All I can do is question, support and wonder at what my clients' come up with and then achieve.

Oh, and one last thing. This is very active work – *you* have to do the work and the more you can do between sessions, the greater your progress will be."

Harry sat dumbfounded for a moment. Well, he thought. I have signed up for what sounds like hard work! If I am going to do this, then I might as well, for once, put my all into it!.

Turning to Mary he said "No magic pill and all's well then?"

Laughing, she retorted "Unfortunately, and although many clients' have wished it, I don't have a magical cure."

In that case, "Let's get started! Where do I find the library?"

Chapter 3:
The Library

Harry walked with Mary down the wide Entrance Hall, his feet padding softly along the polished wooden floor. To either side of the hall were large doors, most of which had brass door knobs and finger plates that looked exceedingly old.

"How old is this place?" he asked Mary

"As old as you are expecting it to be."

"It reminds me of some old gothic manor house."

"Then that's what age it is."

They carried on walking for a short distance, until Mary stopped outside a door.

"This is the library. As it is your first visit, I'd like you to keep your mind open to anything that may or may not be in there.

Setting Intent

First however, I'd like us to set our intent about what you will do with, gain from, or achieve by this experience."

"What do you mean 'set my intent'?"

"Oh, sorry, have not I talked to you about that yet? I meant to mention it before we came here. In that case, let's put that right straight away.

Setting Intent is all about voicing what you wish to accomplish by doing or participating in something, prior to starting it. Intents should always be stated in positive and present terms. For example, my intent for our session today is to help you find out how you learn about yourself."

Let's set our intents for this room you are about to visit. How would you like to start?"

"Do you mean something like, 'My intent is not to find anything that might hurt me"

"That's pretty good for a first attempt, but think about what words you have used. What you've said is that you 'don't want to find anything'. Do you think that would help you learn about yourself?

"No, I suppose not"

"Try and rephrase the sentence so that it is more positive."

"How about; 'My intent is to find out about things that will benefit me and be good for me'."

"Excellent! You've picked that up really easily. So, I'll set my intent now. My intent for bringing you here, is that you begin the processes of self-healing, self-discovery, self-development and self-learning."

Having set his intent for going into the Library, Harry wondered what it was that might not be in there that he would miss, but kept quiet about that idea and just agreed that he would keep an open mind.

Mary gestured for him to open the door and go in.

"Aren't you coming in too?" he asked

"Not for a while, this is your room, spend as long as you like in there. I'll come in if you ask me to, otherwise I'll wait out here for you."

Harry grasped the door knob and turned it with a mixture of excitement and apprehension. He was aware that he

was rather... what was it? Worried, scared or both, he
turned the knob and pushed the surprisingly heavy
wooden door open.

A library with a difference

As he stepped into the room, he was amazed at how dim
it looked and how dry the air was. As his eyes adjusted
to the light levels and he began to notice what the room
was like.

It wasn't like a normal room with four flat walls. It
seemed to have two side walls, but the wall that the door
was in and the fourth wall seemed to create a sort of
curved shape at either end of the room.

Along all the walls were dark wooden shelves. Some
contained what he took to be books; others had large
gaps in them, or were totally empty. In fact, there were at
least three-quarters of one wall with no shelves.

Harry walked up to the far end of the room where the
shelves looked like they were groaning under the weight
of books. As he approached, he realised that they
weren't just normal books that he might find in his local
library. What he had taken for books at a distance turned

out to be beautifully bound covers with lots and lots of different coloured pages inside them. He picked one out at random. The title read 'First Day at Nursery School'. He began to flick through the pages which were also titled. He read such things as: Upset; Abandoned; Happy; Sleepy; Hungry; Tired; Playful; Unsure; Comforted; Really happy; Content; Loved. As he got to the end of the book he found pages of pictures that obviously related in some way to the title and still further on he found some pages that had small indents on them that said 'press here'. He pressed one and immediately the room was filled with the shrieks, laughter, crying and shouting of a nursery school.

He pulled out another book this time with the title 'Three Months Old' and opened it to find similar pages inside. This time, as he flicked through he found: Frustration; Hunger; Pain; Tiredness; Sleep; Affection; Love; Hunger; Bloated; Sleep. Again, he found pages of pictures at the end of the book and yet more pages with the indents that said 'press here'. Just out of curiosity he pressed one. He heard a baby crying. He pressed another and heard the sounds of someone murmuring to what he presumed was the same baby. He pressed yet another and heard slurping noises that reminded him of listening to his own children feeding when they were babies.

Harry moved to a different area of the library and pulled out another bound set of pages. The one he had chosen was entitled 'Stag Night'. Again he flicked through the pages and found: Anticipation; Fun; Laughter; Irritation; Annoyance; Calm; Laughter; Rudeness; Hunger; Thirst; Bloated; Need a loo!; Laughter; Drinking; Laughter; Drinking; Laughter; Drinking; Bloated; Lots of Fun; Need a loo!; Hot; Hotter; Drinking; Laughter; Light Headed; Drunk; Loss of balance; Laughter; Blackout! Quickly Harry flicked to the back of the book for the pictures but there were only a few, and obviously taken early on in the evening. The sounds page however told a different story! Wow! That certainly sounded like a good stag night! He vaguely wondered what had happened to the pictures.

He pulled another book from a different shelf. The title was 'Senior School – First day of term, 1976'. Flicking through the pages in this book, Harry was surprised and slightly worried by what he found: Indifference; Boredom; Frustration; Loneliness; Anger; Surprise; Belittlement;

Ignorance; Hurt; Revenge. All the pictures in this book were tinged with a grey fog like effect; Harry wondered why. Then he got to the sounds page and played a few back. Oh, how awful that sounded. Teenagers goading each other, being rude and derisory. How kids could be that hateful to each other he would never know.

He put the book back where he had found it and turned to look over at the blank shelves and wondered why they were empty. However, he noticed there were not as many empty shelves as there were full ones.

He walked back towards the door, opened it and asked Mary to come into the room. He walked over to her and sat down.

'What can I help you with?" she asked

Harry at first wondered what he should say in response to such a direct question, but instead, launched into the words that seemed to pop into his head.

Life's events

"My first impression was of lots of books, but they're not like normal books. They're separate coloured pages that are wonderfully bound as well as sheets and sheets of pictures and a weird sheet that when you press sections of it, plays back some kind of recording.

The pages seem to be life events that are from really early in life through to more recent things that have happened. I am not sure why there are gaps left on shelves or whole shelves without anything on them. And, there are fewer shelves without anything on them than there are with bound books on them."

"Have you thought about what this room might represent?"

"Well, I am guessing that it has got something to do with my life, otherwise I wouldn't be here."

"Correct. And what do you think might be represented in here?"

"Well, each book seems to indicate a specific event or day in my life, but the pages inside didn't really make any sense, because all they had on them were individual words. Looking at the pictures might help a bit because I might recognise something or someone, but some of the sounds that went with the events made the hair on my neck prickle and stand on end."

"Let's just concentrate on the words for a moment. What sort of words were they?"

"Well, things like: frustration, laughter, anger, hunger, sleep, love or drunk!" said Harry laughing

"And what sort of words are they?"

"Descriptive words."

"Yes, now take that idea and expand it. Think about what the words are describing."

"They describe various emotions or feelings. I suppose, if this is all my life, then they're feelings that I must have had."

"Perfect!" exclaimed Mary. "You've got it exactly. This library holds all the events that have been significant for you during your lifetime so far and records all the emotions, images and sounds associated with each event, so that you have references to remember it by. Some, like a great meal, may even have taste and smell."

"But what about the pictures that were all foggy? And the blanks along the shelves? And the fact that there aren't many shelves left completely empty? And why do all the different emotions have different colours?"

"Wow, you have become curious! Let's take your questions in turn and see what you can find out about yourself.

Did you notice anything about the colours of the pages in each of the books?"

"They're all the same colour for the same emotion or feeling."

"Great! So what can you deduce from the range of predominant colours in your books?"

"Oh dear. Most of them were quite dull. Greys, dark blues, greens and purples. Lots of 'sludgy' colours."

"And what has that told you?"

"I guess that most of my emotions are negative, depressing or dull."

"Has that been true your whole life?"

"No. There used to be lots of oranges, reds, yellows, bright blues, greens, pinks and white and lots of bright and pastel colours, but all that seemed to change towards the end of my senior school and into university, and well, the drab colours have taken over now."

"So, what can you learn about yourself from the colour changes in your books?"

"That I need to lighten up! That I want to start having fun again. That I have to find things that'll help me be more positive about life in general. I'll just make a note of those."

⇒ Lighten up!
⇒ Have fun!
⇒ Be more positive about life!

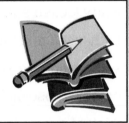

"Those are three excellent starting points. Let's get back to your original questions again. What about the gaps on the shelves?"

"I'm not really sure. I suppose there could have been years when I didn't have many significant events in my life."

Mary sat nodding encouragingly, so Harry carried on.

"But what about the lack of shelves? Surely there should be some?"

The future

"I must admit, that is quite unusual. There's normally a full wall of 'future' shelves with at least one or two books on them. The only reason that I can suggest for not having anything there, is that you have made no long term plans for your future."

Harry looked aghast. How could he not have made plans for himself and his family? He must have planned something! He sat and thought for a moment, but nothing, absolutely nothing, came to mind. He tried to think of events that were on the calendar at home, but he couldn't recollect anything. He hadn't even thought of booking a holiday for this summer!

He was sure the children had all sorts of things planned, but his wife dealt with all of that!

Guiltily he admitted that no; he didn't have any plans for the future. He hadn't even written a will! Something that his financial advisor kept trying to get him to do, but that he just couldn't see the point of at the moment. He wasn't old enough to die!

"But why are there so few shelves left empty then?" he added.

"That's something I have often seen. All I can tell you is that the number of shelves seems to indicate how long you currently expect to live."

Harry was visibly shocked that he had so few shelves left, but Mary continued

"However, what I would like to emphasise, is that the shelves in this library have a habit of changing in all sorts of ways, such as the number of shelves and how many books are on each shelf. And they always change for the better!"

Harry made a mental note to book some holidays, plan a party for his wife, organise a fund for his kid's further education and start thinking about all the good things he and his wife would do after his retirement.

He was brought back from his thoughts as Mary was speaking and he had already missed the first sentence of what she said whilst he was thinking about his will.

"… get you to think about and write down at least three goals that you would like to achieve in the long term.

Let's say, 5, 10 and 15 years time. They can be as
adventurous as you like, in fact, write down your dreams!"

⇒ What are my dreams?
⇒ 5 years
⇒ 10 years
⇒ 15 years

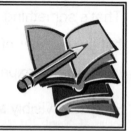

"I would also like you to think about what you've learnt in
this session about the way you remember your past and
how you are living in the present. Concentrate on the
various colours of your emotions and think about how you
can make changes in your everyday life, starting right
now, to think in a more positive way about everything.
Finally, I would like you to set an intent for each day.
Don't worry if something doesn't seem to go quite right,
just set a new positive and present intent each day.

You have a lot to take in from today and to be getting on
with over the next few days, but I am confident you are
already learning and will easily take it in your stride."

And with that, Mary moved towards the door, indicating
that this session was over.

Harry followed Mary out down the Entrance Hall and to the seats where they'd first sat and chatted when he arrived. He felt both tired and elated, as if something was already beginning to shift, although he wasn't sure what. He thanked Mary and agreed he would see her in 10 days time for his next session.

As he walked back to his car, he felt a spring in his step that he hadn't felt in ages. He smiled as he passed a couple of young mothers pushing prams; he even noticed that the birds were singing in the trees.

Yes, this was definitely the right thing to be doing for his health.

PART 2

HOW DO WE COMMUNICATE WITH OURSELVES?

The thoughts we think and the words we
speak, create our experiences

(Louise L Hay)

Chapter 4:
The Study

Harry met Mary again, wondering what would happen this week. Last week had been amazing. He was still reeling from learning so much about himself.

They said hello, exchanged some pleasantries and did a quick review of the previous session in the Library.

Harry looked through the notes in his book – he had added a lot since last week.

"I have achieved loads by just reflecting on previous events, I have learnt how to see different perspectives and be more positive. That comment about lightening up has been running around in my head all week. I have also realised the value of setting intent for the day, it gets me really focused on the important things and seems to work!

"What was the best thing about your session here last week?"

"That's easy! I got to be part of the whole experience and really understand how I had constructed my Library and how it was relevant to my life."

"So, what do you feel you have learnt from that experience?"

Harry took a little time to think over what he had done at the previous session in the Library and read out the following from his notes:

⇒ I enjoyed being part of the whole experience, so that's something that helps me to learn.

⇒ Everything I encountered last week had been relevant to my way of life now and for the future, so relevance was important too.

⇒ I wasn't really aware of being 'taught', but I certainly learnt a lot. Mostly about myself. So I am not really sure how that fits in, but I know it is all part of how I like to learn.

⇒ I realised the value of reflecting positively on previous events – I suppose that is learning from the events that happen to me."

"Now that you have a few examples of how you learn, would you like to find the Study and discover what you really *do* know, what you think you know and what you don't know that it would be helpful for you to learn, or become aware of? I am sure in the process, you will find out what you enjoy most about learning and what style of learning suits you best.

And before you rush off, would you like to set your intent?"

"I have been doing it every morning and I have already done this morning's. Do I have to do another one now then?"

"Well, it is useful to set one every time you embark on something new. They don't have to be just one-a-day things."

"Oh, I hadn't realised that. I have only been doing them once, will that matter?"

"That is fine and let's also set one for today's part of your journey. Would you like to go first?"

It wasn't a question, so Harry thought for a moment, before saying, "My intention for today's session is to enjoy the way I learn about learning."

"Excellent and my intention is to help and guide you in your learning."

Harry still wondered how much more he could possibly learn today, but he had enjoyed the last session so much, that he put his doubts to one side and went wandering off down the ornate hallway towards a set of doors at the far end.

As he walked, his eyes adjusted to the light and he began to notice pictures on the walls of varying sizes that he hadn't been aware of before. Some were huge dark, dingy looking portraits of what he presumed to be old masters of the house or 'learned men' of some kind. Others were what he thought of as 'abstract', or 'modern art', for they were not discernable pictures of anything, but blocks of colour in sizes that went from about A4 size up to well, he wasn't sure how big, but they'd certainly have covered his lounge walls at home! There was one in particular that caught his eye. It was a large painting, he would guess about the size of a door, hung horizontally. He thought at first, it was a picture of the sea, but when he went closer to it, he realised it was different shades of blue, with a white line separating them. He looked for the small card that would tell him what it was called. 'Study in Blue' it said, but there was no artist's name.

He turned and walked on. Passing a couple of doors on his left, he tentatively tried the handles, but they were locked shut. He started to walk on, but something caught his eye on the other side of the hallway. He did a double take, for he was sure he was seeing things. Across the hallway was the painting he had admired earlier. This time the blue picture was hung like a portrait and reached all the way down to the floor. He checked the label. 'Study in Blue', just like the other one.

As he moved towards the picture, Harry noticed that what he had thought were just two blue blocks of colour, were in fact lots of different shades of blue, progressing from really pale at the top of the picture, to deepest blue, almost black, at the bottom. As each shade changed, there were bumps and ridges in the paint and as he stroked his fingers down the picture to feel the difference in shades.

As he reached the middle of the picture it suddenly gave way and moved back away from him, causing him to fall forward. He panicked, thinking that he had destroyed the picture. Then realisation suddenly dawned on him.

The picture had given way, because it was the entrance to the Study!

What Harry finds out

How could he have been so stupid! Fancy not realising that the title of the picture had been a play on words and that he had passed the entrance to the Study once before! But then, how could he have known that is what it would be?

Harry stood still for a moment looking at the blue picture door. He wondered 'is this my first lesson? Is this how I will learn?'

Straight away, he sat on the floor and pulled out his special notebook. In it he wrote…

⇒ The lesson is not always in the form I expect it to be
⇒ Withhold all preconceptions about how I think I learn
⇒ Be open to new ways of learning – however bizarre they might seem

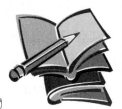

Then he got up and walked a little further into the room and spotted Mary sitting in an alcove. He vaguely wondered how she had got there before him, but decided not to say anything about that, so instead said, "Even the door has taught me that if I don't learn the first time, the same thing may just appear slightly differently next time."

"Harry, just think about those pictures you saw in the Library of you taking your first steps – how did you learn to walk?"

"I really can't remember, but I do recall my children learning to walk.

First they learnt to crawl, they made so many attempts but they never gave up. They made all sorts of mistakes; they tried arms only, they tried legs only and I can remember one time my daughter got onto all fours,

picked up her arm and toppled over onto her back
instead of going forward; both of us just burst out
laughing and she was giggling too. Then, when they
were trying to stand up there were the dozens of times
they just collapsed onto their bottoms and started all over
again. But once they had taken their first steps, within a
few days they were walking naturally without a second
thought."

"So, if learning anything maybe similar to the way you
went about learning to walk, what does that tell you about
how you learn?"

"Let me see," Harry counted off the points on his fingers
as he said them:

⇒ You learn more when it is **fun** or interesting.

⇒ **Mistakes are fine,** they're just feedback to try something different next time – don't give up.

⇒ Don't keep repeating the same mistakes, because you will get the same results.

⇒ Progress is gradual – **a gradient** – babies go through stages of crawling etc., before they try to walk and become expert.

⇒ Seeing parents walking around on 2 feet and cheering when you succeed is just the **inspiration/motivation** you need.

⇒ When you get it right it quickly becomes a **learnt skill.**

"And is that reflected in how you learn today?"

"I'm not too sure. The idea gives me an apprehensive feeling, but I'll try to work it through:

Fun – Learning at school was a hard slog and certainly not fun. But I suppose I had to learn lots of stuff then. Learning about myself with you now really is fun. There seems to be no end to how much fascinating stuff I can learn – I see why people say personal growth is a lifelong journey.

Mistakes are fine – Ha! Try telling that to my boss! I get scared to do things that I think might work and terrified of taking any form of risk, because he will make such an issue out of any mistake made. So I quickly learnt that lesson – not to be creative and use my initiative – that is one of the reasons why I hate my job. And it is not just the mistakes; he makes people feel as if they are really stupid and I don't want to keep being made to feel bad about myself.

A gradient – The event that springs to mind here is when I tried to re-tile the bathroom – a simple DIY job for most people or so my wife told me. And she did expect perfection first time. Guess what, I got really frustrated because it wasn't going right, made a terrible job of it, lost my temper and had to call in a professional in the end. What did I learn from that? Well I still hate DIY so I don't think I learnt a lot. But maybe if I had taken baby steps, read up how to do it, talked to my mate Dave (he's a builder) and started with a small splash back above the toilet basin, it would have been a different story.

Inspiration/motivation – I need to see progress and that is exactly what I am seeing here with you. I know I can do this with a bit of guidance, because I have seen changes already. And I have started noticing things in other people too – my happiest friends are also the healthiest. It is such a simple thing but I would never have noticed without you suggesting it. You get inspiration from within yourself as you start to believe that you really can do something to create better health.

A learnt skill – Things can so quickly become automatic. I remember when I learnt to drive; it all seemed so complicated, but by the time I took my driving test it was much easier and now I seem to drive almost on "autopilot." I don't remember all the gear changes I made to come here today. But I have noticed that bad things can become automatic too – that packet of crisps at lunchtime, a cigarette in the car and snapping at the kids – they have all become automatic."

"Brilliant!" exclaimed Mary, and she handed Harry a small sheet of paper with the following diagram on it, that fitted exactly into his notebook.

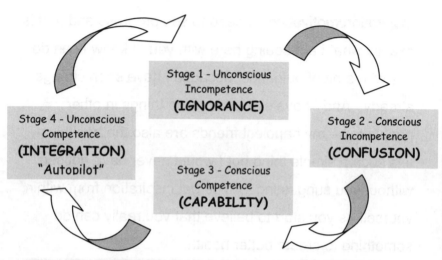

"This diagram is a way of expressing what you've just realised. It might help you in the future, so I suggest you keep it in your notebook for reference purposes.

It is amazing how learning to walk can give such a great metaphor for other types of learning too. You may notice there were no manuals to teach you how to walk, no walking lessons; you just experimented without fear of having to be right. Once you had the skill, it was easy to do for the rest of your life, without a second thought."

Creativity

"Whilst you are here, I should like you to briefly consider your own creativity."

"Oh that's easy; the boss says I never have a creative thought!"

"But you are a designer, is that really true?"

"No, but any idea I have is either squashed or he takes it for himself."

"Could you just think for a moment about the creative process – how do you get your ideas?"

"Oh, I get you now. Sometimes they just pop into my head, at other times, when I get stuck, I look through the relevant information and then take a walk; ideas just arrive."

"That is great and also a great model for talking with your subconscious or unconscious. Just think about the question you have in mind and relax. Trust yourself. An answer will always come to you and you don't have to try too hard to achieve this. In fact, the less you try, the easier the communication.

The most amazing piece of creativity is the development of the baby in the womb, the mother does not decide to 'make a leg today', she just allows space for growth. In the same way you can just allow space for your growth and space for you to develop your own method of communicating with yourself and listening to your own wisdom."

Positive Intent

"Before we move on, could we just check back to that section that you called 'Mistakes are fine'. Your boss doesn't seem to agree. So tell me, what do you remember from when you were a toddler?"

"One thing I am still perplexed about is the amount of 'No's' I gave my kids as toddlers, so I am guessing I had the same. Can you explain why everyone is and presumably was, so negative? It seems to be that learning to walk was fine, but the minute kids master that, it is almost as if we as parents had rather they hadn't. So again, I am guessing I went through something similar when I was a toddler."

As Harry finished his sentence he immediately heard the following ring out in his head:

'Leave it alone!' 'No, put it down!' 'Yuk, dirty, let go!' 'I told you not to touch!' 'no, No, NO!' 'Put it back' 'No, be

careful!' 'I told you you'd hurt yourself, come here,
Mummy kiss it all better'.

"Oh that one is quite easy to explain. They're all phrases
your parents used when they were trying to protect you."

"Protect me?   It didn't sound much like protection."

"That's because they weren't overtly telling you they were
trying to protect you. They were using what's called
'Positive Intent'. Although it looked and sounded like they
were telling you off, their Positive Intent in doing so was
to protect you from harm. Lots of parents sound like
they're telling their children off, but if you can take a step
back, look at the situation and understand the parent's
motive, there is generally a positive intent behind what
they're saying.

Let me give you an example. Many parents use the
simple phrase "I want, doesn't get." Their positive intent
is to teach their child to ask for things nicely, as in 'please
may I have', but all the child hears is that whatever they
want they can't have. Some children completely forget
how to 'want' and then only have goals they 'don't want' –
that should sound familiar; and you will understand how

this doesn't help us in the longer term; but the parent's intentions were good."

Harry thought about how he had spoken to his kids, and often still did. He might shout at them to not do something, but he was trying to teach them how to behave or how to do something safely. Now he understood what Mary meant, he would certainly change the way he said things. Maybe that would make for a more peaceful life at home too, because the kids would understand why he was saying what he was saying.

Harry brought his attention back to Mary as she continued.

"Behind each action there is always some kind of positive intention. Imagine the following actions; getting to work, feeding the family, getting the children to school. Now, think about what the positive intentions behind those actions are; the more you ask yourself what your positive intent is for an action, the more likely you are to get back to some very basic human instincts. For example, survival, protection, nourishment, safety, learning and personal growth.

Although it doesn't seem like it to you right now, your boss may be trying to protect you in just the same way."

"I would never have thought of that as an explanation for his behaviour. And it may take some time to get to grips with this in relationship to him, but I will give it a try.

That's something else I have learnt today then. I'll just make a quick note of that before we carry on."

⇒ There is always an underlying positive intention to every action

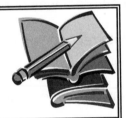

A new perspective on learning

So, now that you know there are lots of things that you don't know, you don't know, what will you do about it?"

"I can start to find out what they are. I can make sure I am open to new experiences and new ideas. I can experiment with things I have never tried before. I can look for differences in the way I do things that might bring about a different result."

"Oh, excellent work, Harry. You are on a roll now. So what will you do if someone or something gives you a negative response, or doesn't work for you?"

"That's O.K. too. I can take a step back from whatever the result is and just take it as feedback. I don't have to take everything people say or the way things work out so personally. If something doesn't work out, then I can try a different way of doing or saying it."

With recognition of what he had just learnt, Harry said "That's how I spent my years as a toddler learning. It was only when I got to school that I started being told I wasn't any good at things or that I should try harder, but at school I never got positive feedback about things that went wrong, only negative feedback, so I just gave up. Well, all except for art and design, which I guess is why I am doing what I do today."

"So, what do you think of what you've covered today?"

"Oh it is great! I can see myself changing all sorts of things over the next few days. Mostly at work; I'll just have to keep taking steps back and trying to find the positive intent of my boss! It should be easier at home though."

"On that note, I think we'll call it a day then. I'll look forward to hearing all about what's changed next time we meet."

Chapter 5:
The Sound Studio

Harry arrived for his session with Mary and was looking forward to a calm and quiet session. He had been working hard over the last week or so on a project for a high profile client. It had been his daughter's birthday during the week, so his wife had been stressed with organising ten little girls for an afternoon and had been sniping at him! As if he could have told the client it wasn't convenient to work this week! Added to that, his brain was in overload with constant chattering. It had been going nineteen to the dozen with suggestions, counter-suggestions, arguments for and against and all about such trivial things. He could do with sitting in a quiet room and just relaxing. He hoped that was about to happen.

Mary greeted him at the door as usual and asked how he was. Before he could even sit down, it all came rushing out of his mouth, faster than he could think about it. He regurgitated everything he had been thinking about in the last few moments.

"Oh, that sounds quite a lot to be hearing in your head"

"Yes, it is. I wish it would shut up. I can't hear myself think! I am amazed I didn't have an accident on the way here! It was like having a car full of people, all in my head."

"I know you said you'd like quiet and calm today, but, how do you feel about tackling all these voices in your head? I am sure you could make a bit more sense of things if you understood what was going on and why."

"Right now, I'd do almost anything to get them to quieten down, or preferably, go away!"

"In that case, I think it might be prudent for you to visit the Sound Studio today."

"Sound studio? Do you have a recording studio here then?"

"Not exactly, why don't you come and explore."

With that, Mary rose from her chair, which was an indication that Harry should follow her into the Manor House. He got up and walked up the Entrance Hall.

Now, where would a sound studio be? He had often heard of rock stars having studios in their Manor Houses, but he had no idea whether they were in the house itself or somewhere in the grounds. Mary stopped slightly ahead of him and turned around.

"Before we go any further, let's set our intents for this session."

"Oh, yes. I almost forgot. I have been doing them and often more than one a day." Harry paused for a moment and then said "My intent for this session is to understand what all the voices in my head are doing there, how they might help me and calm them down."

"That's a lovely intent. Mine is to guide and direct you so that you will enhance your learning of how the voices can and do help you."

With that, they both continued down the hallway.

Harry was on the look out for doors with strange names as he walked, but it was the sounds of someone shouting

that guided him towards the far end of the east wing hallway and one particular door.

As he approached the open door, he could hear a man's
voice shouting. Incoherently at first, but the closer he
got, the more he was able to make out what was being
said.

He pushed the door open to reveal a comfortable looking
room that was nothing like he imagined a recording
studio would be. As he looked around the room, he
noticed huge fat chairs with pairs of earphones draped
across their arms. At one side of the room were two vast
mixing tables with lots of knobs and buttons and fader
panels on them and dotted about the floor on stands
were microphones with giant lollipop style mouth pieces
on them. Otherwise, it looked like a really comfortable
lounge, although unlike a normal lounge, he noticed there
were no windows in this room.

How does Harry speak to himself?

Mary and Harry sat down in two of the comfy chairs.
'Maybe he was going to get his relaxation after all'
thought Harry.

But Mary pressed a button on a remote control by the side of her chair and to Harry's surprise the man's voice started shouting through what he assumed were hidden speakers, and he sounded quite angry. The voice said:

"You stupid idiot!"

"How could I have forgotten that"

"What did you go and do that for?"

"Call me 'Mr Potato Head'!"

"Oh god, I am so stupid!"

"You're never going to succeed at this"

"What a plonker!"

"Why didn't you finish that at work?"

"Why did I buy such an expensive house?"

"You really should give up smoking"

"Just one more biscuit"

"It is only a couple of pieces of chocolate"

"Oh, for heavens sake, what were you thinking of?!"

"You clumsy oaf!"

"Fancy forgetting to bring it"

"Like, I'd be able to do that!"

"I'm dying for a fag!"

The voice continued with lots more negative comments for a couple of minutes more, until Harry put out his hand, grabbed the remote and pressed STOP.

"OK, I have got the message, that is me and those are just the sorts of things I think to myself all day long. No wonder I get so fed up and down about everything."

He sat back in his chair glad of the enveloping support and continued "That is a dreadful way to speak to anyone. Hearing all that, I am just hurting myself and I am not even noticing it. And its not only what I am saying, it is the nasty tone I am saying it in. Does everyone speak like this to themselves?"

"Not everyone, but you'd be surprised at how many people use some or all of the phrases that you use on yourself. You'll be happy to know that you are not the worst, nor the best client, I have known come to this room."

That made Harry feel ever so slightly better, but not much.

"So have you any ideas about what affect all this self-talk is having on you and your health?"

Harry had never given how he talked to himself a second thought, let alone think how it might affect his health. He wondered how he could give himself a worse time than he gave his enemies – well, people he didn't particularly like; they weren't exactly enemies. Did he really have such a low opinion of himself?

"Actually, I have never even considered that what I hear in my head might have an affect on my health"

"I thought as much. Let me just tell you about a study that was carried out some time ago.

Research done in the 1970s by Dr. Ronald Grossarth-Maticek surveyed 3,055 elderly residents in Heidelberg, Germany and generated an attitude rating that scored between 1 and 7 (7 being a very positive attitude). The percentage still alive and well 21 years later varied from only 2.5% of the people with scores of 2 or less, to 75% of the people with scores of 6.5 and better.

"Now, where would you like to be in that survey?"

"Well, obviously at the 6.5 or above level. Wouldn't everyone?"

"What the people with an attitude of 6.5 or above did, was unconsciously, take responsibility for their health and by simply having a *positive* attitude. It doesn't matter whether we are being negative to other people, or just to ourselves. We hear both the same way, as our subconscious is always eavesdropping on our every comment, whether it is spoken or just thought and the essence retained. So, if you can suspend judgement of others, you stop judging yourself."

Having listened to Mary, Harry wondered why he had never heard any of this before; but then he realised he was being negative again! Just by not knowing something that someone else did, who had promised to support and guide him. There was no reason for him to have known about that research. So, he consciously made a decision not to worry that he had never heard it before, and just be glad that Mary had told him about it now.

Knowing now that his subconscious would pick up every thought, whatever it was, he realised it would make a difference to his life. He had been and certainly still was at the moment, feeding his subconscious much more negative talk than positive talk.

Harry made a note in his notebook. It was taken from the Walt Disney movie, 'Bambi'. He had always remembered this little phrase, but never actually thought about it in relation to himself before now…

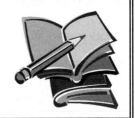

⇒ "… If you can't say somethin' nice, don't say nothin' at all…."

Mary explained. "We all have an internal dialogue, or self-talk, with ourselves that helps us sort out situations. All manner of discussions take place inside our heads." For example, just sit quietly for a moment and imagine hearing the words *you have won the lottery*."

Harry's mind was instantly flooded with voices telling him what to do with his winnings.

Mary went on. "Whilst all the voices in our heads mostly sound like us talking to ourselves, some of the voices belong to other people in our lives, all we have done is taken on their 'personality' and the type of things they'd say, but under the guise of our own voice. These voices are sometimes known as 'introjected voices'. All that means is that they're someone else's ideas or values that we have taken on as our own with our own voice. They're normally picked up early in life, from people in authority, or people we look up to, or trust. Do you know the sort of people I mean?"

"You mean like parents, or teachers or older family members?"

"Yes. That's the sort of person. Why don't you listen again and see if you can identify any introjected voices. If there's one that's particularly dominant, we can do some separate work on that later if you would like to."

Listening in a different way to what was going on in his head now, Harry was sure he could hear his mother saying 'give it to charity" and his father saying 'invest it', whilst his football friends were suggesting that he buy a life-long season ticket for them all and his wife was telling him to 'pay off the mortgage'.

Mary continued, "This internal dialogue is with you 24 hours a day and is a very natural process to help you make decisions, resolve situations and plan actions."

She asked him to listen again to the type of discussion going on; he could even hear his answers to various suggestions and sometimes he got into a whole conversation and even an argument with himself!

Mary asked him to notice whether these statements were positive or negative and to see if he could tip the balance to being positive.

Harry dutifully sat and concentrated on all the conversations going on in his head. He had to admit that, most of them would be classed as negative. He tried to change a couple that he was having with himself and immediately succeeded in doing so. He tried the same thing with what he thought was the voice of his mother, but that didn't seem to work very well. What she was saying still sounded negative. He tried another of his own conversations, instant success again. What if he tried the one that sounded like his wife that was going through his head. That had slightly more success than his mother's, but it wasn't a complete change or, as instant as when he was talking to himself.

He made further notes in his book.

⇒ Positive self-talk is more beneficial to my health

⇒ Change what I hear and how I hear it in my head

⇒ Introjected voices are often early programming from other people.

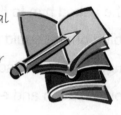

Should's, ought's and try……

The next thing Mary asked him to think about was how many times he said out loud or, in his self-talk, the words "should" or "ought" – and notice how it sounded.

"Actually, it sounds quite judgmental."

She then asked Harry to think for a moment what the word 'should' actually meant to him and the feelings it generated.

Harry heard a familiar sentence run through his head.

'…You should have finished that, but you have not; you failed again…'.

"Oh no" he groaned "And its one of my most used expressions. It is as if I am talking down to myself. I am judging myself all the time and the answer is failure." It even gave him a sinking feeling in his stomach.

Harry realised that every time he said 'should' it signalled failure. He had been trying to give up smoking for years. Just thinking about it now, there was that voice... "You should give up smoking..." Harry realised that it wasn't his voice, but someone else's saying that to him, who was it? It sounded like the sort of thing his wife said regularly. And the more she told him to give up, the more he resisted making any change at all. If only he had his own voice saying 'I will give up smoking because I want to', how much more empowering that would be? It would be his own decision when and where.

He sat back in his chair, he was learning so much so quickly, his head was in a spin and what is more, he knew he had heard all this talk all along, but had never for a moment thought to sit down and think about just what he was doing to himself.

His mouth was very dry, and his legs felt stiff. He got up out of his chair and strolled across the room to the water cooler, then wandered around the room drinking. As he did so, he wondered about the sounds he had heard in the library that were associated with the coloured pages of emotions. Had he been talking to himself like this for ever? No, not forever, but probably since senior school! Hey, here he was doing it again! But this time, it was useful information that he was working out. This was going to help him move forward in a more positive manner. Now that he was aware of what he did, he could do something about changing it. Feeling better about himself, he walked back to his chair and smiling at Mary, told her he was ready to go on with the rest of the session.

Going around in circles

Mary suggested they explored how Harry used his internal dialogue.

Harry told Mary how some of his internal dialogue seemed to be like a stuck record. It would just go round and round repeating itself, with him feeling he could never move on. His internal voice presented the same arguments and the same options, and to his surprise, he would always get the same answers.

It was particularly bad at night, when he tossed and turned for ages, going through all the things that had happened during the day and then once he had gone through all of that, he would start on what it was that was keeping him awake and what he could try to get to sleep.

"You'll learn how to deal with that issue when you find the bedroom. However, until that time, I'd like to make a suggestion that will help see you through until then."

So Harry made a note…

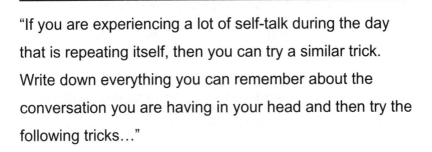

> ⇒ Write everything that's in my head down on paper before going to bed.
> ⇒ Turn over and close my eyes. It will all be there in the morning.

"If you are experiencing a lot of self-talk during the day that is repeating itself, then you can try a similar trick. Write down everything you can remember about the conversation you are having in your head and then try the following tricks…"

As Harry listened to Mary, he thought these were great ideas, so he wrote them all down in his notebook and decided to try them out over the following few days.

⇒ Imagine jumping forward six months, is the problem still a problem, or has it faded away?

⇒ Sit in a different seat and look across at what I've written. (looking at the problem from a physically different perspective can help find a solution.)

⇒ Give two of my friends or colleagues a copy of what I've written. Then, ask them to sit either side of me and fire their own questions at me about the problem. (They should both talk at the same time, so that my conscious brain can't reject any ideas and they can all just seep into my unconscious.)

"Let's have a short break and then move on to another subject that is reflected in your self-talk or internal dialogue."

Harry got up and wandered around the studio, stretching and bending as he walked. He pretended to be a rock

star standing at the microphone with one headphone
over an ear, the other just behind his other ear and his
finger pressed against the ear without a headphone on it
– just like he had seen on documentaries about music of
the 60's and 70's. He noticed Mary had taken a different
seat, so he did too. Hmm, just changing seats made
everything in the room seem different.

We like to be right

Mary asked Harry if he liked to be right.

"Well, yes. Doesn't everyone?" He couldn't imagine
anyone not wanting to be right. Not deliberately.

"There's a well known NLP saying that goes… 'If you
think you can, or you think you can't, then you are right'."

Harry thought about that for a moment. Basically, if he
thought he could do something then he could and he was
right. If he thought he couldn't do something and then
didn't achieve it, he was proved right too.

"So, if I think I am going to have a good meeting with a
client, I will. But if I am not looking forward to seeing a
client and expect the meeting to go badly, then that's
what happens."

"Exactly so. Everyone unconsciously supports the behaviour that confirms their expectations."

"Let me just tell you another example, so I know I have got this right."

"O.K. Go ahead"

"If I am trying yet again, to give up smoking, but I don't really believe I can, then I won't be able to give up. Even though consciously, I am trying to.

"That's it. You've got it."

"Whoa, that's quite bizarre. I mean, that I can be thinking I am doing one thing, but actually, I am making sure I am right and sabotaging myself, so I don't succeed."

"It is the way the unconscious mind works. As I said, it likes to be right."

She carried on. "When we have internal dialogue or self-talk, we also generalise things. That is to say, that if one thing is true of an issue or event, then it is true for every other occurrence of that same or even a very similar event or issue. So, if I was to ask you if you knew of an example where you generalise, would you be able to give me one?"

"I think so. It is something that gets me quite annoyed really. I am convinced that my boss is always late into the office; so even on the very rare occasion that he might be on time, I'll unconsciously ignore that time and just remember the times he's late, because they support my generalisation about him being late, all the time."

"That's a perfect example. I am guessing that actually he's not really late that often, it is just that you are now so convinced of your own generalisation, which you unconsciously delete the times he gets into the office promptly."

"And there was that time that the media latched on to the theory that people who wore 'hoodies' committed crimes. They had then proceeded to make such a big thing of it in the press and on TV, that it was almost accepted as a national generalisation that everyone who wore a 'hoodie' was a criminal. It was clearly not true, but the way it was put across was enough to worry many people on the street and I remember some shopping malls took the, in my opinion, extreme action to prevent 'hoodies' being worn by anyone inside the mall, despite the fact that some of the shops were actually selling them!"

"I think you've got the idea of generalisations. I'd like you to start listening to yourself as you speak or as you self-talk and just become aware of when you are using generalisations yourself."

"OK. I'll just make a note in my book, so I don't forget what we have just talked about, because there was a lot in there."

⇒ The unconscious always likes to be right. So, if I think I can, or I think I can't, I will be right!
⇒ The unconscious doesn't do negatives
⇒ The unconscious deletes things that don't match my generalisations about people and events.
⇒ Change from saying 'should' or 'ought' – they don't help me!
⇒ Who are my introjected voices? (work on those with Mary later, if I want)

"Would you like another break? I just want to set up another voice clip; I'll only be a couple of minutes."

"Sure, I'll have a wander around and choose a new seat."

Mary came back from across the room where she had been doing something on the mixing tables.

"Ready? Let's hear them then."

And with that, Mary pressed another button on the remote.

What do we say in metaphor?

This time the voice wasn't Harry's, although it sounded vaguely familiar somehow. He started concentrating on what it was saying.

"I'm dying for a break"

"My feet are killing me"

"I'm feeling so full, I could burst"

"Just the thought makes me feel sick"

"He makes my skin crawl"

"I just turn a blind eye"

"It is enough to make my hair fall out"

"You'll turn me grey"

"I'll never make old bones"

"They'll be the death of me"

"It makes my stomach turn"

"He's deaf in one ear"

"She makes me sick"

"I can't see for looking"

Mary stopped the playback. "Can you hear what is being said?"

"Well, I heard what was said, but they're just normal phrases that everyone uses."

"Yes they are, but if you remember, we were saying earlier that the unconscious always likes to be right, so it takes these phrases literally."

"What, you mean it tries to make someone sick, or their eyes go blind?"

"In a sense, yes. The unconscious will do what it can to facilitate our wishes.

I know of a story one of my NLP teachers tells about his mother. She had recently gone through a lot of upheaval in her home, her family had grown up and left the house and she had been working really hard in her nursing job.

She kept saying that she was "dying for a vacation." She was diagnosed with breast cancer."

"Oh my god. You mean it can be something that serious?"

"That's quite an extreme example, but things like that do happen. What I'd like to know is whether you have a 'pet metaphor', like those you just heard, that you use frequently, which could be affecting your health."

Harry sat thinking. He couldn't think of anything he said like that. Not on a regular basis anyway.

So Mary said, "Why don't you try a body scan? Imagine you are looking at your body from inside and think about every part of your body; just see if anything gets highlighted for you."

Harry sat back and let his attention slowly pass from one area of his body to another. When he came to his elbows he said "I do have a bit of itchy rough skin on my elbows, but I have had that for about 3 years, could that be something to do with a metaphor?"

"Is there anyone who came into and has been part of your life for the last 3 years who really gets under your skin?"

Of course, it was his boss, Harry exploded, his face going bright red as he spoke. "It's my boss. It has to be – I may not say it, but I often think that he does things deliberately to get under my skin!"

"Just a moment. Firstly, is that the message you want to keep giving yourself? And secondly, this is *your* reaction to him, you have a choice, you don't have to let him get under your skin. Can you think about him differently? Do all your colleagues think of him like this?"

"Well, no. Not all of them. Although there are quite a few who feel like me."

"So, how could you think about him differently?"

"Well, I suppose, rather than him getting under my skin, I could just dismiss him as a waste of space!"

"Even that's better than how you started, although I think you could probably change that idea too, if you tried."

"He's actually pretty incompetent and if I set my mind to it, I could do his job really easily."

"That's much better. Can you make that sentence shorter or more succinct?"

"I can almost feel sorry for him! Good grief, how did I get to this? Anyway, to answer your question, I think I'll just look at him and feel sorry for him, because I know he's not up to it."

"Great. Now, how long did that take?"

"A few minutes."

"And you've managed to go from causing your health to be effected, to feeling sorry for the person who was the original catalyst. How good is that?"

"Pretty good I suppose."

"I'd say that was excellent! Well done. Now you know, just spending a few minutes changing how you think about an issue, can change the whole perspective and its impact on your health. Can I presume that you will do this from now on?"

"I will certainly do my best to change whatever I am thinking to something that won't hurt me, or that's more positive. Does this mean that this itchy rough skin will go?"

"It will just take a short while for your unconscious to change its programme, so that it is right. Assuming there are no other motives or reasons for it to stay like that, I am sure you'll notice a difference within a week or so."

"Phew, that'll be a weight off my mind" said Harry, and then laughed at how he had slipped into using a metaphor straight away.

"In fact, that brings us nicely onto the next subject in this room."

Affirmations can create change

"Have you come across affirmations before?"

"No, what are they?"

"An affirmation is a positive sentence or phrase that you repeat on a regular basis. They are very powerful in support of changing current life patterns and behaviours for new ones."

"So, just by saying something positive to myself, I can make a change?"

"Yes, saying it on a repeated and regular basis is the key to affirmations working. So, as you are changing how you talk to yourself about your boss, you might have an affirmation that reflects your change in attitude."

"What, something like; 'my boss can't get under my skin'."

"Not exactly. They should always be stated as if you are already experiencing the desired change. And if you get internal dialogue along the lines of 'you have to be kidding', or 'this is not real', or 'yeah, right!'; just acknowledge that you heard it and remind yourself that the reason you are doing this is for a change to occur or become a new habit. If you can repeat your affirmation thirty-three times a day for thirty three days, it really becomes a part of you."

"You've been using negative thoughts for almost all your life, so changing them is not going to happen overnight, but if you persevere, you'll get there. I suggest you start with some simple ones and go from there."

Mary proceeded to take Harry through the process of creating an affirmation and as it was new to him, he made some notes in his notebook.

⇒ Write down what I want in life
⇒ Create positive statements from my 'wants' list
⇒ Write in the present tense, as if I am already experiencing the affirmation's content
⇒ Never mind the self-talk 'back chat'
⇒ NO negatives!

"So, will you create some affirmations and bring them with you next time you come please. I'd like to make sure that you've got everything in the correct tense and that you are associated into the statement."

"Associated into it?"

"That just means you can really feel, see, hear and experience what the affirmation is like. As if it is real life already."

"O.K. then. I can do that. I'll write them all in my notebook, so that I remember to bring them with me."

"Excellent."

Listening to his body too

Now, we have talked a lot about what you hear in your head, but we have not touched on how your body communicates with you, to tell you something's wrong. What do you normally do if you are body tells you something in the form of a small ache?"

"Ignore it! I just take pills to take the pain away and get on with my day."

"Oh, I see. Knowing what you know now about communication, do you think that's always a good idea?"

"I suppose not. It might explain why I get lots of aches and pains. I am just ignoring whatever my body is trying to say, aren't I?"

"It would rather appear so, yes. What change could you make that would make a difference to how you respond to your body?"

"You know in the Study, I learnt about positive intent. Well, does my body have a positive intent with these aches and pains too?"

"Yes it does."

"In that case, I could try and understand what the positive intention of the ache is and when I find out, I could make a change to whatever is causing it."

"That would be an excellent change to make. It also shows that you are integrating what you've learnt from previous sessions, into your daily life, which is great. So, do you have any aches or pains at the moment, or perhaps you've had some since our last session that you could explore now."

"Well, I have had an on and off headache for over a week."

"That would be a good example to use. What do you think all those headaches were trying to bring to your notice?"

Harry knew all too well. He always got headaches when he was really pushed for time, stressed and had too much to do, but he said. "That I am trying to achieve the impossible; like all good Supermen."

"And what can you deduce or surmise or learn from the message of a headache? Remember, it is all about you getting the signal from your unconscious as to what that particular part of you wants you to consciously do."

"It's probably trying to tell me I have taken on too much, or that I am spreading myself too thinly."

"Rather than just guessing at what it is trying to tell you. Can you relax, put your attention onto the headache and wait for a message to pop into your head?"

"Don't know. I have never tried that. I guess you want me to try it now though, eh?"

"If you are willing to, I am sure it will help you understand how you receive messages from your body. You are in a very safe environment here, so no one is going to comment on what you do, say or experience."

Harry sat back in his chair, closed his eyes and took three deep breaths, allowing his body to feel like it was sinking back into the chair. Then he thought about the last time he had had a headache, where in his head it had ached and how it had felt. He didn't think anything was happening and was about to open his eyes again when he heard a voice in his head say 'too much stress', 'need to delegate more', 'trust other people to do the work', 'do what I am good at.' Startled, he opened his eyes and sat bolt upright.

"I presume from your reaction, you just got a message?"

"Err, yes. I think so. I wasn't expecting anything and then all of a sudden I heard this voice in my head telling me things."

"And did what the voice say make sense to you?"

"Yes, unfortunately it did, every word. In fact, it is almost like it knows me better than I know myself."

"That often happens. Remember, you are working with your unconscious here. It is going to know things about you that may not be in the realm of your conscious mind yet. Has what it said helped you understand the reason for the continuing headaches though?"

"Oh yes. It was very eloquent!"

"Good. So now that you know their cause, you can make a change, or some changes and benefit from no headaches and a new perspective on their cause."

"Yes, but what if I don't understand the message I get or I get no message at all?"

"Ah, that's another question that comes up quite often. You will have to trust that your unconscious knows what it is trying to achieve and that it can communicate with your conscious mind so that it will understand, even if you don't think you do. If you really have no idea what's going on, then you could always ask your unconscious to try giving the message another way. Perhaps as a dream, so that when you wake up, you understand the process and the outcome of the change to be made."

"Oh, so I can have a sort of conversation with this voice in my head, just like if I am talking to myself in internal dialogue?"

"Absolutely, the more you can communicate with different parts of your body as well as your unconscious mind, the more benefit you will get from these messages."

"So I could have a conversation with this rough skin on my elbows and tell it that I have sorted out the cause and that it is O.K. for it to clear up and go now?"

"A perfect example."

"Oh, I didn't realise I could do that. Does everyone do that?"

"Unfortunately not, mostly because they don't know they can. They're still in the situation you were before today's session. They don't know that they don't know, that they can communicate with all parts of their body and mind. You have just moved forward quite a few steps in your self-awareness."

Harry smiled shyly and fidgeted in his chair. He liked being told he had moved forward, or achieved something, but it didn't feel comfortable yet. He wondered if it ever would. But right now, he would just let the warm glow he was feeling inside spread out over his chest and across his arms and legs.

"So, now that you know what to be aware of, you can start to get more insight into both your self-talk and your body's messages. They can both offer you wisdom that you cannot consciously be aware of, so I would strongly recommend that you have daily conversations with them. Perhaps do a body scan in the shower in the mornings, or check in with your body before going to sleep and if you are experiencing lots of internal dialogue what are you going to do?"

Harry flicked open his notebook:

⇒ Write down the challenge
⇒ Physically move and look at it from
    somewhere else
⇒ Ask friends of colleagues to help
⇒ Even see what I might learn from the
    situation

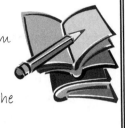

"Excellent. I think you've got all that settled in a positive frame of mind. I think we have about covered everything there is for you in this room. Is there anything you'd like to go over, or ask me?"

"Can I just write down some notes and check them with you before we leave?"

"Of course."

So Harry opened his notebook and wrote, even repeating some of the things he had already written down, but that didn't matter because it would help him really get it into his conscious brain.

⇒ Be positive – focus on what I want
⇒ Be as nice to myself as I am to others
⇒ Careful of metaphors – my body may take them literally
⇒ Support myself in everything I say to myself or others.
⇒ I like to be right so reinforce positive messages.
⇒ take some positive action
⇒ Be positive about achieving whatever I set my heart on
⇒ Eliminate words such as *should*, *ought* and *try* from my speech.
⇒ Suspend my judgement; I don't need to judge myself
⇒ Be optimistic, it is more likely to happen.

"I think that's an excellent list Harry. I can already hear how much more positive you are in your thoughts. Just keep at it and it'll become so natural, that hearing anything negative will seem odd to you."

"Is there anything I should do between now and our next session, other than practice what I have learnt today?"

"No, I think you'll have quite enough to be getting on with for now. I'll look forward to hearing the affirmations you come up with at our next meeting."

And with that, Mary rose from her chair and led Harry back via the Entrance Hall to her front door.

"Thanks Mary, I'll see you in another 10 days or so. I'll work really hard on all this."

And with a wave, Harry walked back to his car. As he got in he thought, 'I sound different already!'

Chapter 6:
The Drawing Room

As Harry arrived to see Mary, he was wondering what today's session would bring. He clutched his notebook as he wanted to tell Mary the affirmations he had created since his last session in the Sound Studio.

Mary greeted him and asked how he had been. Harry was very proud of himself, as he had been repeating his affirmations every day, often at least 3 times in a day. He wasn't sure if they were working yet, but he was certainly feeling a lot more positive about everything. Even his boss!

"Congratulations. That's really good progress. Is there anything you've thought of that you'd like to go over again, or have questions on from your last session?"

"No, I think I am all O.K. with that thanks."

"So, have you given any thought to what you'd like to address in today's session?"

"Well, no not really. Is there anything that follows on from what I did in the Sound Studio?"

"As you explored the sense of sound last time, do you think it is appropriate for you to explore another one of your senses and how it can work for you?"

"Oh, that sounds good to me. Which sense?"

"We, or rather you, can get to know your visual sense this session, as it will follow on nicely from your work with affirmations."

"Is there a special room for the visual sense then?"

"Of course, but remember, it will be specific to you and how you learn and what you have to learn, so I can't tell you where it is."

"OK, I'll go and have a wander through the mansion and see what room opens up. Will you be coming with me, or shall I meet you outside again?"

"That's entirely up to you. What works best for you?"

"I think I'll go in on my own and call if I think I need you. Shall I set my intent here, or when I find the room?"

"Let's do them here, so that we can set them together."

"O.K. then; my intent for today's session is to carry on the learning I started in my last session and enhance that learning wherever I can."

"That was really good Harry. Your intent's are getting more focused and you are more aware of what you want from these sessions. That is excellent progress on both fronts. My intent for today is to assist you if you get stuck, with options that allow you choice and growth."

And with that, Harry left Mary at the seat in the Entrance Hall and headed off to the hallway of the mansion.

Finding the right room

He wasn't quite sure what he was looking for, but knew by now that he would find the right room. He just had to firstly find and work out the clues that would lead him there.

As he walked, he looked around for anything that might point him in the right direction. At first there was nothing, so he kept walking and as he did, his foot slid on something. Looking down, he noticed an array of coloured pencils on the floor that lead up the staircase. He picked them up as he followed their trail up to the first

landing and along it, turning first left and then right. They
stopped abruptly outside a heavy opaque glass door,
engraved across which was the title "The Drawing
Room", in old fashioned copperplate.

Harry had always thought a drawing room was where the
family of the house had entertained their guests, so he
wasn't sure how it would fit in with his visual sense.
However, he pushed open the door and looked around.

The chairs in here were much more formal than those he
had sat on in the other rooms that he had visited and
there were vast areas of floor space, covered by piles of
paper, blank canvases, pastels, crayons, paints and inks.
There were even some piles of clay in one area.

Harry sat on one of the chairs and looked around him.
Apart from the floor space there were large areas of the
walls that seemed to be divided up into sections and
covered with picture frames containing blank canvases.
Harry though it rather strange, that anyone would hang a
blank canvas, but maybe it was some kind of modern art.

Pictures of the mind

As he stared at one of the sections, a picture began to emerge on the paper, as if by magic. He rubbed his eyes – he must be more tired than he thought. But no, it was definitely there when he looked back at the space. As the picture became more complete, Harry was surprised to see the road he lived on and his house in the middle, except his house had been freshly painted, just the colours Harry had been thinking about last weekend.

He turned to another space on the wall and again, a picture started to emerge. This time it was of his family when he was still a young kid; sitting around the dinner table, enjoying a roast dinner. How he used to love Sunday roasts when he was a kid, and lamented the fact that now, his family very rarely had them. The kids always seemed to eat first, and then he and his wife would eat on trays in front of the TV later in the evening. He had often imagined how the scene would look in his own house of them all sitting around the table for a Sunday roast, and as he recalled that vision, the picture changed in front of his eyes, to his imagined vision of his own family.

He looked in a different direction and began to think about all the illnesses he had had so far that year, which had brought him to this point. Immediately, a picture started emerging on the blank canvas, but not a very nice one. He saw a bitter and sick old man, coughing and wheezing in a chair, all alone in a room that looked dull, very dreary. Harry imagined that it probably smelt damp too.

What a horrid picture. Who was it? He was sure it wasn't anyone he knew. He turned and focussed on another blank picture frame. This time he thought about how he would like to be in 6 months time. There appeared on the canvas, an image of Harry, but not the one he had seen in the bathroom mirror this morning. This one had clear skin, bright eyes, looked like he had lost at least a couple of stone in weight. He was smiling a lot too, and looking at all those people who were being friendly towards him. Who were they?

Harry really wasn't too sure quite what was going on, but he had realised that he could see images, which he was thinking about, appear on the blank canvases.

He looked back at the areas of floor with the piles of papers and canvases and drawing materials. Then went over to one of them, sat down on the floor and imagined a tree. As he got an image in his head, he began to pick up the pastels and paints and draw the image that came to him, just as he was imagining it. He didn't care what colours he was using, or whether the tree was true to life, he just sat and drew. When he thought he had finished he looked at what he had done and was quite surprised. In front of him was a tree that looked like it had just been plucked from the wild wood. The trunk was short and gnarled; the branches twisted and blackened; the roots spread wide, but were very shallow and it was painted in really drab colours. Harry wondered what had got into him, to create such a dull, drab picture. He was sure he had been thinking of something bright and light and full of life.

He moved back over to one of the formal chairs and focused on a blank picture. This time he put all his energy into imagining what he would be like when his kids got married, that was a good 20 or so years away. He was expecting to see a sprightly 60-ish year old that would follow on from the version of himself in 6 months time, but instead he saw the wizened, sick old man he had seen before. What was going on here?

He decided to go and get Mary. She would help him sort this out, because he was sure things in this room weren't working like they should.

Harry asks for help

"Hi, how's it going?"

"That's why I have come down to get you. I thought I was doing O.K. and understanding what was going on, but I have just had a couple of surprises that I don't think should have happened and I'd like you to come and help me sort them out please."

"Sure, lead the way."

Harry explained what had happened as he led Mary back to the Drawing Room.

"... So, you see, I should have seen this sprightly 60-ish year old, and instead I got that grizzly old man come up again. So, I think there's something wrong with the room, because it is not bringing up the right pictures."

"That's very unusual. It is normally 100% accurate. Are you sure you think you'll be a sprightly 60 something?"

"Well, no. Not exactly, but I'd like to be."

"Ah, that's where the picture is getting confused then."

"What do you mean confused?"

The focus is on your belief

"Well, if you can't really imagine yourself being a sprightly 60-ish at your children's weddings, then what the pictures will show you, are your hidden worries of what you think you might really be like. The impact of pictures that we show ourselves, can be even more powerful than the internal dialogue we run."

"You mean, I think I am going to be that grizzly old man?"

"No, I mean, you are worried that that's how you will turn out, and that worry, or negative thought, is overriding all the positive images you are giving yourself.

Remember in the Sound Studio we talked about the more you think of a negative worry and therefore 'hear' it, the stronger it becomes? Well, the same happens for images too. The more you worry about how something might turn out for the worse, the stronger the image becomes, and the more you imagine that image, the more energy you give it and so it becomes a stronger vision. That overrides anything more positive, that you don't unconsciously truly believe.

Visualisation is one of the easiest tools to use and can have one of the most profound effects on your health and well-being, beneficially as well as detrimentally, if you visualise the 'worst that could happen' or even 'what might happen' scenarios. That's why it is important to repeat your affirmations, so that your unconscious believes them and can create the visual image to go with them."

"So can I change my negative images in the same way as my negative self-talk?"

"It's a similar way, not exactly the same."

"So, how do I do it then?"

Changing to the positive

"You're quite lucky, in that you don't have any problems with visualisation, so I'll just skip to the part about how to change. However, if you are going to explain this to anyone else, you might want to put these notes in your notebook – just for reference."

Harry took the notes and scanned through them. Yes, it all seemed perfectly straight forward to him. 'How could people not understand how to visualise?' Anyway, he stuffed them into the back of his notebook, because you never knew who you might bump into and what might be useful one day. *(See Appendix 2 for Mary's notes on how to visualise)*

Mary continued… "You have good visual skills; you are used to using them for your work and imagining out into the future what a particular piece of work will look like."

"Yes, I can bring a whole project to life in my mind"

"Our personal experiences of life are enormously enhanced by having a great visual memory – the trick is to keep it positive and focus on what you want, not what you don't want."

"Where have I heard that before?"

"My point exactly. People often worry about things that may never happen. If you've had a bad experience, or you want to change a negative worry that keeps popping up as a particular picture; here's what you can do."

Harry hurriedly got out his notebook and wrote as Mary told him how he could change his pictures.

How To Change A Negative Visual Image
⇒ Change the picture(s) from moving, to still
⇒ Change from 3-D to 2-D
⇒ Change colour to black and white, or sepia, or even fade it out to almost nothing (white on white)
⇒ Move the picture back from you, so it becomes smaller and smaller; it can even disappear into the distance.
⇒ Put a frame around the picture
⇒ Remove any sounds you hear that are associated with the picture or, change them into a ridiculous voice, such as a cartoon voice

---

"Now, give those ideas a try with your image of the grizzly old man and see what happens."

Harry did so, with some remarkable results. "Hey, it is going! This is amazing."

"Good, now what do you want to replace it with?"

"Me being a sprightly 60-ish."

"In that case, imagine your picture of yourself as being the sprightly, 60-ish, father of the bride or groom and reverse all the suggestions I made earlier, making the image better and better. Add in as much detail as you can to the image you want, including feelings and sounds."

Harry started to create his image of how he thought he would look, adding in colour, movement, sound, smells and feelings. He made the 2-D image into a 3-D one and changed the picture from a 'still' into a movie. He took away the frame and expanded the size of the picture so that it filled the whole of the wall opposite his seat. As he was imagining the picture, he felt he could almost jump into it. He told Mary what he was doing as he changed his image.

"What you've done is excellent. The only thing I'd recommend is that you don't bring your picture too close, otherwise you might overpower yourself. Keeping it at

arms length, or maybe even a couple more feet away
from your body, is the closest space I'd recommend."

Harry made a quick note below the previous ones...

⇒ Never bring my picture closer than
   arm's length away from my body –
   it may become too overpowering

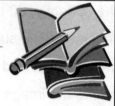

"It's that easy?"

"Yes, it is that easy. Just focus on imagining what you
want to do, or have, or be, rather than what you don't
want.

Positive visualisation has been known about and used
extensively in sports for years. In Linford Christie's book,
'To be honest with you', it says he always visualised
himself breaking the tape, and winning the race. There is
also a story about Linford and Colin Jackson doing all the
preparation for the gold medal celebration before the race
– they did everything to visualise exactly what they
wanted."

"Oh, wow. In that case, I think I'll try a few more of the
blank pictures here in the room to see what comes up, or

maybe have a go at drawing or painting a future that I'd like to happen. Oh, that reminds me. I painted this tree. What do you think that might mean?"

Mary looked at the tree. "It strikes me that this is how your unconscious might think of you at the moment. Have you asked it?"

"Oh, I forgot about the conversations with my unconscious. Do you think it is a message?"

"I'm not really the person who can tell you that. Why don't you sit quietly for a few moments and have that conversation with yourself. I am sure you'll find out far more by doing that, than having me make suggestions about my interpretation of your drawing."

So that's just what Harry did. He found out that at the moment, his self perception was not very positive or healthy and that had been reflected in his drawing. So, now he knew.

Practicing moving to the positive

He also knew that if he drew the image of the tree that he wanted to become, he would have a much more positive image to work towards. He thanked Mary for helping him and asked if it would be O.K. to stay in the room for a little longer.

"Of course, you will know when it is time to come back to the Entrance Hall seat."

So Harry stayed in the Drawing Room. Moving about the room, watching excitedly as the pictures on the walls emerged and then using the techniques which Mary had taught him, to enhance or fade them. He drew pictures of what he wanted, making them bright and big, and using lavish strokes of the brush or pastels. It was when he tried to draw another picture and realised that he had used up all the papers and canvases that he understood it was time to go. He wondered what would happen to his pictures if he left them here, so rather than not know, he gathered up the ones he was really pleased with and took them with him back to the Entrance Hall.

What Harry learnt

Mary was waiting on her seat and looked through his pictures with interest.

"These are wonderful. They are truly inspirational and I am sure they will help with all your visualisations of what you want. What else did you learn about visualisation?"

"Well, I realised that I can do it easily. So, I think I am going to use it more than the affirmations I created following our last session."

"What if you were to combine the two practices? What impact do you think that might have?"

"I suppose I could. I just thought it would be easier using the one I am best at."

"Yes, it would be easier, but is that all you want?"

"I'm doing it again aren't I? I am letting myself down because I can't be bothered to try something that's not easy. No, you are right. I will combine them. After all, I was pretty good at conversations with myself too!"

"As with the affirmations, I'd like to hear, or perhaps see, what you decide are your most important visualisations at our next session."

"Oh, I can tell you that now. It'll be me in 6 months time, looking and feeling fit, healthy and happy."

"The key is to visualise and affirm these things as if you have them now, so maybe bring your visualisation forward and look at it as an ongoing state of health and happiness over the next 6 months."

"Oh, yes. I forgot. I'll do that then. An ongoing state of health and happiness it is!"

"Is there anything outstanding that you'd like to ask me about today's session?"

"No. I am really pleased with myself today. I have had a great session and I can visualise all sorts of things that I want."

"Remember Harry, only positive things. Never, ever, visualise something negative happening to anyone else, for it will surely come back to you."

And with that, Harry thanked Mary for the session, arranged his next appointment for two weeks time and left Mary at her door.

Walking back to his car, Harry started to notice how bright colours had become, how shafts of light and shadow danced beneath the trees as he walked along. He was looking forward to the rest of his day.

Chapter 7:
The Ballroom Of Beliefs

After catching up with Harry since his visit to the Drawing Room, Mary suggested they go straight to today's room. Harry was a little surprised, but followed her anyway because it was unusual for her to be so directive and so he guessed that there was a special reason that he should visit this new room today.

As they walked up the stairs and along the first landing, Mary asked Harry whether he had any strong beliefs about the world, the universe or life in general.

Without a moment's hesitation, Harry replied. "Well, I certainly believe that we only get one chance at life, so we have to make the most of it."

"And are you making the most of it?"

Harry thought for a second or two, before answering. "I liked to think I was, but I know sometimes I was just pretending that everything was great. Since I started working with you I am becoming more and more aware that I probably have not up until now. However, since I have been exploring all these different aspects of myself, I am beginning to change the way I think and maybe that will change what I believe."

Mary smiled and went on in silence, allowing that thought to settle with Harry as they walked.

They approached a pair of enormous double doors that reached fully from floor to ceiling. Mary stopped outside. She turned to Harry. "This room is one of the largest rooms in the house and one of the most amazing."

"What room is it? What's inside then?" asked Harry

"To answer your first question is easy, it is the ballroom. Your second question, I can't answer. That will depend on you. Everyone who goes in comes out with a different answer about what they find inside. I have not met one person yet, who had exactly the same experience in this room as any other. Would you like to set your intent before you go in?"

"Oh, I totally forgot that. Um, well, as I don't really know what I am going in to, I guess it'll just have to be, 'to learn with grace and take on the lesson'."

"And my intent is to be here to support you in your learning."

Inside the Ballroom

Totally intrigued, Harry turned the handle of the door. Although heavy and solid, it swung open with surprising lightness and ease. Harry walked inside and heard the door softly click shut behind him.

He stood for a moment taking in the scene. The room certainly was huge. From where he was standing he could see a balcony at the other end of the room, on his left were panelled walls covered with gilded mirrors, a really high ceiling, from which hung massive chandeliers whose light danced and sparkled off the mirrors. There were floor to ceiling windows that ran the entire length of the right wall and overlooked the gardens of the house and heavy brocade curtains held back by twisted golden rope ties hung at either side of the windows. There were delicate gilded chairs in small groups around the room, and the wooden floor was polished with such a shine that he could see his face in it.

Harry realised that he was just standing, staring around the room in amazement. Then as he stood there, he began to notice other things about the room. Like the plasterwork that was painted in gold and the palest blue he had ever seen. Wow, he thought, how intricate and delicate that is. And what a detailed pattern there is in the floor, but all in blocks of the same wood – clever. He suddenly stopped himself looking around with the shocking realisation that he would never normally notice anything like that. Up until now, a room was a room, was a room.

Lost in his own thoughts about what he had noticed, he became aware of a sense within himself of the room being physically empty and yet so full that he was almost being jostled as he stood still. It was as if the room was full of people dancing around him and he was in their way.

He moved over towards one of the mirrored walls. He would be out of the way here.

The mirrors tell stories

As he walked towards the mirror he was astounded to see a reflection of not just himself, but of various scenes from his life. He rubbed his eyes, thinking he must be tired, but when he opened them again, the same images were showing in the mirror. They seemed to be depicting snapshot scenes from when he was a small boy, through his childhood years and teens, even into and through his 20's and 30's.

He stepped closer to the mirror and examined a few of the scenes more thoroughly. Yes, it was definitely him, and mostly including his older brother too. There was his brother being given a bike for passing his 11-plus, getting a cup for playing rugby, being a prefect, getting his degree, getting the offer letter for his first job, getting married and at some awards dinner. What was it with his brother being in all these images? Wasn't this supposed to be all about him, not his brother!?

Harry felt really resentful that his brother was in his images. His brother was always good at everything he did, always came first in games and sports, always got the best job and had the best life! 'Unlike me' thought Harry.

Feeling fed up, Harry turned and looked towards a different mirror. Thank heavens. Just a normal reflection. It was happening again. What was going on in here?

Harry looked hard at the new mirror and was shocked to realise that he was looking at lots of different images of himself. Except that they weren't really him. Well, they didn't look like he looked.

One was a wizened old man with no hair, lots of lines, a pale, sallow complexion and a haunted expression on his face. One was almost comical, it looked like someone had blown him up with a pump, but had forgotten his head, hands and feet. In another he looked as if someone had squashed him with a huge weight, in another he was a cowering, sickly looking about the same age as he was now, in another he was excessively tall and thin like a pencil but a gust of wind kept blowing him over.

Harry turned from the mirror in disgust.

Surely there must be one mirror in this room that would show him something good?

He walked into the room further, passing a couple of mirrors without looking into them, but was drawn back to the next one.

He looked at it, fully expecting it to be as horrific as the last or as disappointing as the first.

At first, he could see nothing unusual, just his own reflection. Didn't this mirror do what the others had done? Then, as he relaxed a little thinking that this might just be a normal mirror, the images started to appear.

Harry took a deep breath, closed his eyes and when he opened them again the mirror was full of images of what he considered to be every-day stuff. There was an image of the night sky with the moon and stars, an image of rain falling from clouds, an image of a simple sum (2+2=4), an image of birds flying, an image of a car moving, an image of hundreds of supermarket shelves! He gave up!

He walked to the middle of the room and looked around. Architecturally, it was a lovely room. He had no idea what else he might or, was supposed to see, but he had had enough.

He opened the huge doors again. This time they were really heavy and difficult to open, not like when he had gone into the room.

Mary was waiting for him outside the room. "How was it?" she asked motioning him towards a sofa on the landing.

"To be honest, a bit mind blowing!" Mary nodded, waiting for him to go on.

"I'm not really sure why I was seeing so many different images in the mirrors. And each mirror showed me different sets of images."

"And was there any kind of link to all the images in each individual mirror?"

Harry sat silently for a few minutes, mulling over what he had seen in each mirror and what it meant to him.

"Well, yes. The first mirror I looked at had all these images of my older brother. They were all to do with how good he is at everything, how successful he is and how great his life is"

"And is your brother all those things?"

"I think he is. He's always better than me at everything."

"And what of the other mirrors you looked at?"

Harry sighed deeply, "The second mirror was pretty awful too. It had lots of images of me in it, but not as I am. They were all distorted in some way.

And the third mirror appeared to have lots of normal, every-day stuff in it. Things that I am so familiar with and take for granted."

"So, with all the work we have done already in mind, what do you think these mirrors are showing you?"

Harry sat staring out into the space in front of him; his head full of what he had seen and how it fitted together.

He went back in time over all the images of his brother, he thought about his relationship with his brother now. He thought about what his brother meant to him.

Then he remembered all the images of himself in the second mirror. He hadn't liked any of them. He had been too fat, too thin, too old, and too ill. Too anything, but not how he wanted to be.

The third mirror didn't seem to make much sense. It was all just everyday stuff. It was stuff that was just, well, there. Would always be there, stuff he knew because that's how it was.

As he sat on the sofa, staring but not seeing, all he could hear in his head was the word 'connections', over and over again.

Harry recognises his beliefs

With a jolt it came to him.

Everything he had seen was connected within the same mirror to what he thought of as true, in fact, it was what he believed was true.

That was it! That was the connection! All the images were things that he believed or that made up what he believed.

Oh no. This was scary. Did he really believe his brother was better than he was? Well, obviously.

And all the distorted images of him were what he believed he was really like at various times.

The third mirror was just confirmation. It was all the things that happen in daily life that we take for granted, but we believe without question.

Harry recounted what he had just realised to Mary, who nodded and smiled as he told of his new understanding.

"So, now that you've learned what this room can show you, what would you like to do with that information?"

"I would like to change some of it. In fact, I would like to change a lot of it. But how does it all get there and how can I change it?"

"I'll explain how it gets there as simply as I can and you can make your own notes from what I say. Then we'll start working through changing one of your beliefs, so that you have the knowledge to move forward and work on your own with others that you wish to change."

Mary's explanation

"Beliefs are important because they have an impact on how you behave.

Let me give you an example: In the 1950's, there was a generally held belief amongst the population that running a mile in less than 4-minutes was not only impossible but, according to doctors of the time, dangerous to the health of any athlete who attempted to do so!

When Roger Bannister crossed the finish line at Iffley Road, Oxford, with a time of 3 minutes 59.4seconds, he broke that belief.

Bannister changed everyone's belief of what could be achieved, (i.e. they had new evidence to add to the images of their mirrors) and therefore, he helped change their behaviour. By the end of 1957, 16 runners had run a mile in under 4 minutes.

Now, let's get back to what you've just experienced.

Imagine that each belief you have is a mirror in the ballroom. When you were born, the mirror would only have reflected you, because at that time, you were not conscious of having beliefs. But, as you grew older, you were told different things that you took to be true because of who had told you."

"You mean like my parents, teachers or I suppose my older brother and sister." Harry paused for a moment, then excitedly shouted "Oh, I get it! So, everything that I learnt, saw and experienced from that point onward supported what I had been told and became an image on my mirror!"

"Exactly. The mirror gets filled with all the images that help you support the belief, and the belief becomes one that you call your own. The more images you have to support a belief, the stronger it becomes."

"And the stronger the belief, the more it becomes a part of who I am. That is what filled each mirror!"

"Right – you have it, excellent work."

Harry was busy scribbling in his notebook...

⇒ When I was born I had no conscious beliefs

⇒ One experience can build or change a belief

⇒ My beliefs didn't necessarily start off as my own ideas

⇒ Beliefs are often handed down from those we look up to

⇒ Beliefs are only as strong as all the images (references) that support them

⇒ Some beliefs are general (the sun will rise in the morning, birds can fly)

"But, how can I change a belief if it has all those images supporting it?"

Changing the belief

"We're just about to come on to that. Changing beliefs is only as hard as you believe it will be. So, what's the first thing that you are going to put in place?"

"Oh that's easy. I am easily able to change any of my beliefs; the process will be easily accomplished"

"What an excellent affirmation of a belief. So, let's work on one of your beliefs that you'd like to change."

Harry recalled what he had seen in the ballroom mirrors. He desperately wanted to change the first two mirrors he had looked at.

As he was thinking which one to tackle first, Mary suggested that if something seems too big to deal with all at once, break it down into manageable chunks or pieces or steps, like the gradient we discussed in the study.

She told him to remember the joke about the elephant that went; "How do you eat an elephant? In small chunks!"

He decided that attempting a whole mirror's worth of images in one hit might be pushing it a bit for his first belief change, so he decided to take just one image from the second mirror, the one that had shown him his belief about himself. Yes, he would change one of those.

He repeated his affirmation about beliefs in a strong loud voice, three times, before he began.

Harry's belief change steps

STEP ONE - Identify the belief to be changed.

Mary asked him to say the belief which the image supported out loud. Much more quietly than he had spoken his affirmation, he said "I always get sick."

"OK. Now let's move on to what you want to change that to."

STEP TWO - Identify the desired belief.

"What you'll do next, is formulate a belief to replace the old one. It must be stated in the first person, the present tense and in positive terms."

Harry sat scribbling in his notebook for a moment. This is what he wrote:

⇒ Always in the first person – I
⇒ Must be in the present tense – "am"
⇒ And always stated positively "
    "Healthy and well"

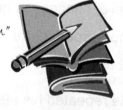

When he had finished writing, Harry looked up and said "I am always healthy and well"

"Great. That's a wonderful belief to have"

Harry was looking puzzled though. He had formulated this great new belief, but how did he make sure it replaced the old one? How would he get a new image for his mirror?

STEP THREE - *Really believing it*

Mary explained that this third step could be broken down into even smaller chunks, so that it made the final process really easy to accomplish.

Chunk one

Harry could use his skills from the Drawing Room and build a picture in his imagination of himself being healthy and well. Once he had the picture, he could add in feelings, sounds, movement, change the picture into a movie and be the star, right there in the movie.

The more often he could run his movie with himself being the healthy and well star of it, the better!

Chunk two

Every time Harry, thought of himself as 'sick', behaved as if he was 'sick' or heard someone else say he was 'sick', he was to stop and immediately replace the phrase used with his new belief. If possible, he was to say his new belief out loud and definitely run his starring role movie.

Chunk three

Each day for a month, Harry was to go through the following sequences:

Run his starring role movie of himself being healthy and well in all sorts of situations and places and with different people.

Say his new belief out loud three times whilst running his starring role movie.

Unroll his ears from top to lobe with his thumb and first finger three times, all the while, saying his new belief out-loud and running his starring role movie.

Do cross-walks (opposite knee meets opposite elbow), all the while, saying his new belief out-loud and running his starring role movie.

Harry tried all these actions whilst Mary was talking him through them and whilst it was fun, it also had an amazing effect on him straight away. He began to feel that he really was healthy and well!

He ended the session with the most enormous grin on his face and promised Mary that he would practice this every day during the coming month.

"So now that you know how to change your belief; on a scale of 1 (being lowest) to 10 (being highest) where do you think you are already, with your new belief?"

"Before that exercise I would have said 1 or even less. Now, I think I'm probably at a 5. This is the first time in my life that I really do believe I can change my health for the better."

As Mary and Harry said goodbye to each other, Harry was now curious as to what else he might see in some of the other mirrors, but that could wait for a while. He already had some other beliefs he wanted to change.

PART 3

THE BIG RELEASE

Energy flows where attention goes

(James Rey)

Chapter 8:
The Lake House - Of Letting Go

Harry returned for his next session with Mary and as he finished telling her what he had achieved over the previous two weeks, she suggested he check out his library for changes, deletions and additions.

How the Library has changed

It was a while since he had started his journey here. He wondered what might have changed over the last few weeks. He opened up the big wooden door and looked inside. As he scanned the room a smile came to his face. A lot had changed. Rather than being dull, depressing and full of sludgy colours, the Library now shone with colour of every hue. There were even lots of new shelves where there had been none and there were even brightly coloured books on those shelves.

Harry rushed back to Mary full of what had changed and updated her.

"That's excellent news. It means that all you've done so far has already had an effect on your health and your life."

Harry sat glowing with pride. This was yet another indication that all the changes he had been making were beginning to pay off.

"Is there anything in particular that you'd like to work on this session?"

"Not especially. I think everything you've been suggesting has been spot on."

"In that case, I'd like to ask you a question that might point us in the direction for today."

"Sure, go ahead."

"Is there any 'stuff' you have hanging around that you want to get rid of?"

Harry looked at Mary blankly. "What do you mean by 'stuff'?"

"Well, I am not sure what it will mean for you. In the past it has meant some or all of the following for various clients: an annoying journey; a dispute with a neighbour;

a misunderstanding in communication; a ticket on the car; someone being sworn at by another driver; rude children; an argument with a spouse; a falling out with a sibling; jealousy or resentment of another person; the list is almost endless."

"Oh, that kind of 'stuff '. That is what my wife refers to as my 'baggage', but does that really affect my health?"

"All of that baggage focuses on exactly what you don't want. So, if you send that message out all the time, what do you think you will get back?"

"Oh, I see. You mean because I'm sending out negativity, I will get back negativity."

"Yes. And what effect do you think that might be having on your health?"

"Oh. I have never thought about that either. I suppose if you are asking the question, then they're having some kind of an effect aren't they."

"Would you come over here for a moment Harry please?"

Harry walked over to where Mary had gestured and stood still as she walked around him turning panels in the wall that became full length mirrors, until he was surrounded by a circle of mirrors.

"Now, try not to move too much and just take a look at these mirrors and tell me what you see."

"Well, I am not as tall as I thought I was, my stomach sticks out, my shoulders are rounded, I am sort of slouching forward and my skin looks washed out."

"O.K., now look past the physical to the metaphor you see and tell me what that is."

"It is someone who can't stand tall because he's got too much weight on his shoulders. Someone who's scared to stick his head above the parapet for fear of being shot down. Someone who has paled into insignificance so they merge in with the crowd and don't get picked on. Someone who is trying to protect themselves with a layer of fat."

"That is very perceptive of you. Let me just expand a little. If you can't stand tall, what happens to your posture?"

"It gets all scrunched up and rounded."

"Yes, and if it is scrunched up and rounded, what happens to all your internal organs?"

"They must get scrunched up and squashed, because there is not enough room for them."

"Exactly! So, can you see now, why it would be of great benefit to release the weight off your shoulders?"

"Oh yes. I see what you mean now."

Harry walked back to where Mary had retaken her seat with a new understanding. He got out his notebook and made the following note.

⇒ baggage effects posture
⇒ posture effects internal organ arrangement
⇒ organ arrangement effects how they work
⇒ solution = get rid of baggage!!

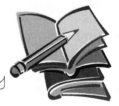

Adding to the 'tool set'

"I have now realised that I am still thinking about things that have happened in the past that are actually quite negative and I sometimes catch myself going over things that have happened in the office say, and wondering what might have happened if I had done something differently, but it is too late by that time and I am just beating myself up each time I do it. I am not doing it deliberately, well, I don't think I am. These memories just pop into my head and when they do, I get a really flat feeling, like something's been taken away and I am just left with an icy cold gap."

"Hmm, that's an interesting description. Are these memories triggered by anything in particular? Like a person, or place, or smell, or some music?"

"I don't know, I have never thought about that. They happen everywhere though, not just in one particular place, although the office does tend to be where I get most of them."

"Is there anywhere in particular that you ache, or that feels tight, or that you have a lot of pain?"

"You mean in my body?" Mary nodded. "Actually, I get a lot of pain at the top of my back and across my shoulders, especially at work. And when I am with my brother, it is like I have gut ache, but it is not really there.

And you know I often get headaches. Why, do you know what is causing the flat feeling and these aches?"

"I have an idea. I would also like you to realise and understand for yourself what is going on and learn how to let go of these memories, or as you have referred to it, 'baggage', because from what you have told me, they don't sound like they are of benefit to you."

"No, I guess they're not. So where do I go to find out about them and how do I get rid of them?"

Introducing the Lake House

"Ah, that will be the Lake House of letting go. It is out in the grounds. You will have to follow the path out of the Entrance Hall and head towards the flower meadow, you'll find it nearby."

"I will set my intent before I go then shall I?"

"That would be good. Then you know you will find the Lake House and easily understand its meanings."

"My intent for this session is to let go of as much as I can!"

"That was pretty succinct! And very positive too. My intention for this session is that you only keep things that are of benefit to you and release as much as is appropriate for you today."

"How will you know if I need you to help me?"

"Oh, I think this session will be pretty self-explanatory, but you can always just call me over, I will hear you."

Harry finds the Lake House

Harry walked off towards the flower meadow, following the directions Mary had given him.

As he crossed the manicured lawns, up ahead he saw a mound of grass full of flowers. That must be the meadow. He guessed the lake was just beyond it, so he lengthened his stride and headed towards the flower covered mound.

As he climbed the meadow to the top of the mound he caught his breath. Ahead of him was a vast expanse of water that stretched as far as he could see. It was surrounded by a flower meadow - well, as far as he could see and beyond that were woods. He looked around for the Lake House and saw it off to the left of the lake. He made his way towards it. From a distance it looked like just a door and a wall, but as he approached, he noticed that the roof was part of the flower covered mound that surrounded the lake.

He opened the door. Inside, the cabin was full of natural wood. There was a really comfortable sofa and chairs, a wood burning stove, photos that had been taken of the lake in various weathers and framed to create a collage and a picture window that took up the whole of one wall, overlooking the lake.

How does this work?

Harry sat down on the sofa and stared at the lake. It was certainly relaxing. He turned and looked at the photos. He was searching for one that might show him what he was supposed to do, but he was too far away, so he got up and walked over to them. Looking more closely at each picture, he noticed that each photo somehow showed the middle of the lake-bed and on the bottom of it was a huge magnet. Harry knew it was a magnet because it was just like the ones he had used in Physics classes at school. A heavy horse-shoe shape that was predominantly red in colour and silver at each open end.

This was all rather strange, but he was getting used to that in his sessions. He went back to the sofa and stared back at the lake. What was the point of the magnet at the bottom of the lake?

He let his mind drift, not really thinking about the answer to his question. Watching the lake ripple in the breeze, seeing still patches reflecting the sunlight, he felt very calm and peaceful sitting there just staring out over the lake. His mind started giving him pictures and ideas; magnets, iron filings, north pole, south pole, drawn together, pushed apart, positive and negative, attraction, displacement, magnetic pull. He let it all swirl through his head as he stared at the lake.

He wondered if there was any music in the cabin. He quite fancied something in the background. He got off the chair and walked around the room, opening cupboard doors. He found the CD player he was looking for, but there didn't appear to be any CDs anywhere. He flipped the 'open' button and the tray came out, with one CD in it. He looked to see if there was a label on it that would tell him what he was about to listen to, nothing. He looked around to see if he could find the case, again nothing. So, he just clicked the 'close' button and hit 'play'. He had no idea where the speakers were, but presumed he would hear something soon.

What he heard was some very gentle music that seemed to have a background rhythm that was almost there, but he couldn't isolate the sound. This would do, just for watching the lake.

Breathe, Relax, Release

He made his way over to the sofa, put his legs up and made himself comfortable. He heard a voice over the music repeating the phrase 'Breathe, relax, release'. Well, it seemed like a good idea, so he shut his eyes, became conscious of his breathing and made it really fill his lungs and then allowed his lungs to completely empty. He felt his back relaxing into the cushions of the sofa, now what was the release bit?

As Harry breathed deeply and became more relaxed, he drifted into that state of being slightly awake and slightly asleep, but still knowing that he was awake.

His mind brought up the various pictures from the collage on the wall. All the pictures seemed to highlight the magnet, which looked like it was getting bigger and bigger in each picture. It was almost pulsating at the bottom of the lake in time to his heart beat, which by now had slowed right down.

Rudely interrupting this wonderful picture, Harry suddenly remembered the fight he had had with his brother all those years ago over who should sleep in the small bedroom and who should have the larger one. What a strange thing to think about. Even odder was the feeling that this memory and the emotions that went with it were being tugged from his chest towards the lake. Eventually it seemed to break free and Harry could swear he saw a wisp of cloud leave his body and head towards the magnet at the bottom of the lake.

He concentrated on relaxing again, only he was interrupted this time by the memory of being dumped by his first girlfriend at school. Again, that tugging feeling came, only this time it seemed to be coming from his knees, and as it finally broke free, he saw the wispy cloud heading towards the magnet in the lake.

Harry was curious about what was happening, but didn't feel like he had the strength or energy to really query or question it. Instead, he relaxed back again, thought about how beautiful the lake was and waited for the next interruption, because he was sure there would be one.

Just as he thought that thought, he got simultaneous memories of two different incidents where he was in an argument about something. He wasn't aware of what the arguments were about, but instantly, he felt a pull leaving his guts and saw the wisps of cloud.

Then even before he could think about relaxing again, memories were tumbling through his head and he could feel little pulls all over his back, followed by lots of clouds going off to the lake.

However bizarre this was, he was just going to let it happen. He stopped thinking anything and just let the memories come up and apparently leave his body. He didn't even try to recognise or analyse the memories, he just let them go.

He started to feel very hot, but the wood burner wasn't on, so it couldn't be that. He opened one eye a bit and saw the sun flooding through the window, filling the room with a golden light that reflected off the polished wood, giving the room an ethereal glow. Maybe that is why he was hot. He swung his legs over and felt a gentle thud as his feet touched the floor.

Noticing what's different

He wasn't sure how long he had sat there, but he felt very rested and refreshed. He stood up and stretched. He felt lighter too, and the pain across his shoulders had disappeared. For no apparent reason he felt the urge to reach down and touch his toes, so he did and surprised himself at his flexibility. He managed to put both hands flat on the floor! He had never been able to do that before! He repeated the motion, just to be sure; yup, flat on the floor. Amazed and feeling great, Harry stood up and turned around to look at the picture collage that had started all those thoughts of magnets. He checked each picture, but as he looked at it, the magnet on the lake bed faded away, as if it had never been there. He became aware that the music had stopped too.

The room was still filled with the warm golden glow of the sun, but Harry wanted to go back to Mary and ask her lots of questions, so he left the Lake House and made his way back to the Entrance Hall where he knew Mary would be waiting for him.

As he walked back towards the main house, he felt lighter, taller and more balanced. His head was high and he was smiling at the day.

Mary greeted him as he walked into the Entrance Hall.

"How was it?"

Questions and answers

"Well, something certainly happened, but I am not sure if it was real or I dreamt it. I think I was awake, but it is sometimes hard to tell in those sorts of situations."

"Would you like to tell me what you think happened?"

So Harry recounted his experience in the Lake House. About the lake that went on forever, the cabin, the pictures showing the magnet on the lake bed, the music, the memories that suddenly started popping into his head, the feeling of them being pulled out of his body and finally about the magnet disappearing from the pictures, being able to touch his toes, not having pain across his shoulders and walking back to her feeling so much better.

"And what, if anything can you learn, or have you learnt, from this experience?"

"Well, based on what I think happened, whether I was asleep or not, but I don't think I was; I can allow my mind to release memories that don't serve any benefit to me."

"Is it just memories that went, or did you feel the power of the magnet attract any negative beliefs, old negative programming, old emotions and limiting beliefs, that no longer benefit you?"

"What do you mean by programming and limiting beliefs?"

"Oh sorry Harry, have I jumped ahead again? Old programming is habits we have developed, without thinking or realising we are doing them. A great example I heard once was about a lady who always cut the knuckle off the end of a leg of lamb before putting it in the oven. It was only when a friend asked her why she did this that she even considered the question. It turned out that she had just copied her mother's habit, who in turn had copied *her* mother's habit. The original reason for cutting the end off of the joint was because the oven was not big enough to take a whole leg in one piece.

Limiting beliefs are those beliefs that we hold, sometimes very close to us, which stop us moving forwards or limit our potential."

"Oh, I see. This time I feel it was memories, but I guess there is no reason it couldn't pull all of that old stuff out of me. It would be great if it could, I am sure I have got loads of that old unwanted stuff clogging up my body. My wife is always saying I walk around with the worries of the world on my shoulders. Although now, I feel like I have shrugged them off - for good! My only worry is that I might lose something that is important to me."

"Don't worry Harry, your unconscious won't let you lose anything that is still important or of benefit to you. It will only release baggage that is ready to go.

Can you remember how to allow the magnet to do its work?"

"I think so. I can imagine being back at the Lake House and seeing the lake outside the window with its giant magnet on the lake bed and then in my imagination I can hear the voice over the music encouraging me to breathe, relax and release. Then I know that the memories that are somehow stored in my body…. Oh, I have just had a thought!"

"Yes?"

The light bulb moment

"That's how I am feeling so much better isn't it." It is because I have released all these negative memories from different parts of my body. That's why I can touch my toes, because my back has become more supple, and why my shoulders don't ache anymore. Oh wow! This is brilliant! I can't wait to see my brother again. I want to see if I get that awful gut ache again, or if that has gone too."

"So, what else have you learnt?"

"That I can just let the memories come out and the less I worry about them, the more I can get rid of."

"Anything else?"

"I have learnt that negative memories are stored in the body and, based on how I am feeling now, if I get rid of them on a regular basis, I'll feel much better physically."

"Excellent work Harry. I'd like to ask you something. Are you aware of having any memories come up that didn't go?"

"Err, no. Not that I can think of. Is that a possibility then?"

"Sometimes a memory, programming or belief will come up and no matter how much we think we're releasing it, it will hang around. It normally means that there is something else blocking its release. That could be some other learning or some positive intent behind it that you have not found yet."

"So what do I do if that happens?"

Using what he already knows

"Think about what you know already that you could try"

Harry sat thinking. He went back in his mind over the rooms he had found already and how they might help him. Then thinking out loud he came up with; "the Library

would only help me find out when or where the memory
had come from if I knew where to look. The Study could
help me be open to learning new things in different ways
or, I could become aware of not knowing that I didn't
know something. Then there's the Sound Studio; I could
have a conversation with my unconscious about it, or the
part of my body where the memory is stuck and try to find
out why it was still there, yes, that would be a good idea.
Now, what about the Drawing Room; I suppose I could
visualise myself finding out why the block is there, then
have it disappearing as I accept the knowledge from it,
that's another option. What about the Ballroom of beliefs
though? What if it was a belief that wasn't really mine?
Well, I could use both of my previous ideas to check that
out and then with all the knowledge I have got I could
release the block that's stopping the memory from going."

"Harry, those are all excellent ideas. I am sure you'll be
able to release and learn from all sorts of memories using
them. However, just in case there's a memory that's well
and truly stuck and if none of what you've just suggested
has worked for you, then may I give you another tip?"

"Of course."

"This may sound a bit strange, but trust me, it works. All you need to do is imagine releasing the block that's blocking the memory from releasing."

"That's it? Why don't I just do that then?"

"Well, you could, but you might be missing out on some insight or learning that is associated with the original memory. Until you get more advanced at this practice, I'd suggest that you stick to the route you've just come up with. The main thing is to keep the process light; don't try to make it difficult or hard, adding in an element of humour to any work you do will help too. The easier you think it will be, the easier it will be. And you can of course, set your intent for that to be true."

Harry took a deep breath. Phew, this was quite a session! He realised he had made no notes at all about anything and was worried that he would forget it all as soon as he left, so got out his notebook and told Mary that he would just like to do a recap whilst he wrote his notes.

"Of course, go ahead."

⇒ Breathe, relax, release
⇒ Let old baggage go to the magnet in the lake
⇒ Baggage = negative memories, limiting beliefs, old programming and negative emotions
⇒ If it is stuck, remember what I learnt in the Study, the Sound Studio and the Drawing Room
⇒ If it is still stuck and I can't get the learning or positive intention, imagine it unblocking anyway
⇒ Negative baggage gets stored in my body
⇒ Releasing negative baggage will help me heal myself
⇒ Imagine sunlight on me as I release the negative baggage
⇒ I don't need to know what's going

"I notice you mentioned imagining sunlight on yourself as you are doing this."

"Yes. That's what was happening to me in the Lake House, so I thought it ought to be on me all the time."

"In a manner of speaking, you are right. What you want the sunlight to do is fill any spaces that have been created by releasing your baggage, with a warm healing light energy. Can you do that?"

"I should think so, it is just a slightly different take on what I thought was happening. I'll make a note so I don't forget."

⇒ When I have finished releasing all my baggage, allow the sunlight to fill my body with soft, warm healing, light energy to fill up any gaps

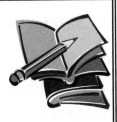

Practice creates self-health

"Mary, how often should I do this?"

"Ideally daily, but at least twice a week if you can. You'll be surprised at how much you can release once you practice this regularly. You will also feel a lot better as the weeks pass and more and more negativity is released from your body's cells."

"Oh, I hadn't realised it was an ongoing thing. I thought just doing it a few times would sort everything out."

"If you keep up the practice, you will release more deep-seated 'baggage' that's either been undermining your health already, or has the potential to seriously undermine your future health. We all take on negativity every day, so if you think of it as a habit to get into, like brushing your teeth before bed, you'll easily work it into your daily routine.

"Why don't we go over to the mirrors before you leave and you can see the difference in yourself that I can already see."

"Oh, do you see a difference?"

"Come and see for yourself."

Harry went back to the area that he had stood in at the beginning of the session and waited for Mary to turn the panels around again, so he was surrounded by mirrors.

Looking at them now, he amazed himself at how different he was from the first time he had stood in this spot. He was now standing as tall as his 6ft 1inch, his paunchy gut had almost disappeared, his back was straight and his head held high. Even his skin had turned a much warmer colour. This was much more how he thought of himself.

"Oh good grief! I can't believe how different I look from when I got here."

"It's pretty amazing isn't it? It also shows you how effective the process you've just learned can be."

"Oh, I'll definitely be doing this regularly. There's no way I want to go back to that awful looking wreck that came in here!"

"That's really good to hear Harry. Just as a post script, if you burp or sneeze or giggle or yawn, those are all really good signs that you are releasing old baggage. And don't be surprised at the affect this might have on your friends and family. I often hear that once someone has started to release their old baggage, it has a knock on affect on those around them."

"Oh, I'm glad you mentioned that, because as I was walking back from the Lake House, I had a sneezing fit. I thought it was because of the flower meadow."

"I think you were probably just getting rid of some cobwebs. Well, unless you have any further questions about your session at the Lake House, I think this would be an excellent place to stop for today."

"Nope, there's nothing else I can think of right now.
Thank you Mary, this was an amazing session, I just feel
so different already!"

"I'm so glad to hear that. And well done you! I'll see you
in a couple more weeks then. Bye for now and take
care."

Harry left Mary at her front door and positively floated
back to his car. He felt so good right now; he doubted if
anything would change his mood for the rest of the day,
maybe even the rest of the week!

Chapter 9:
The ER – Where Traumas Are Dealt With

The next time he visited Mary, Harry positively sprang up the front steps.

He had really been practicing releasing negative emotions, and whatever else his subconscious had felt like releasing. Using the lake and the magnet technique he had seen and felt so much leave his body and he really had no idea what most of it was.

He was feeling a lot lighter and getting nearer to how he used to think of himself (tall, lean-ish, affable, friendly, and happy).

He hadn't had that awful feeling of a muzzy head and total confusion since before his last visit – this was a real result.

Mary asked him if he had noticed whether there were still some negative memories that hadn't been released yet. No matter how hard he had tried.

"Well I think I am doing really well, judging by how much better I feel and it is really fun. Although there is still one issue I can't seem to get rid of. I have tried everything you mentioned last session, but I can't even imagine it going."

"And what is it?"

"I have a phobia about motorway driving. I hate the thought of having to drive on the motorway so much, that my wife has to drive. Meanwhile, I am the most awful passenger. Jenny and I have had so many rows in the car; I hate what it does to us."

"O.K. So when did this start to happen?"

"I was involved in a really bad car crash on a motorway a few years ago. The accident wasn't my fault, but I had to go to court as a witness because someone in one of the cars was killed. I seem to have had to tell so many people the story of what happened, and each time I told it, I re-lived the moments leading up to the crash in slow motion and then again, everything that happened afterwards too. It was horrible. Even now I can feel myself coming out in a sweat and my heart starts racing.

I don't even remember getting home that day, it seems like I was stuck on that road for hours."

"Do you remember when we talked about positive intent? Having a court case pending is a very positive reason for holding on to the whole event in detail and therefore not letting go. It is just that nobody has told your subconscious that the information isn't needed anymore.

It's like the story of the man who caught the big fish – every time he told the story the fish had grown even bigger.

With frequent repetition, over time, the whole incident can become larger than it actually was and that's how your mind keeps remembering it.

Not being able to let go of the incident may also inhibit your recovery, because every time you think of the event you are re-shocking your body.

"I don't think I have ever really fully recovered from it. I would say I am only 50% better, because my neck has clicked ever since the accident.

I had whiplash and when that got better, I was left with this unpleasant clicking and cracking noise whenever I moved my head. My insurance company paid for a year's worth of physiotherapy, but then said I could not claim any more. I still have some negative emotions around that too! It had been a great benefit to me to have an hour per week of 'me' time, which I really enjoyed."

The other thing that often happens is that we all generalise, so something that relates to cars at one moment may in time, can generalise to planes and trains too. We don't *mean* to make things worse; it is just that when our mind generalises, it wants to believe it is true, so goes about proving that it is."

"I get it. With a generalisations I would be trying to find ways of proving myself right – just so that I can justify my belief as correct. I remember that from the Ballroom of Beliefs."

"Well done. Now, let's look at what we have here.

O.K., it sounds to me as if you have 2 issues to resolve here. Firstly letting go, or toning down the memory of the actual event so it isn't so vivid and secondly, resolving your issues around your neck.

"What will this do for me then?"

"It should dramatically reduce your fear about motorway driving, or being a passenger and will start you on the process of allowing your neck to recover.

What I need to check with you is whether you are happy to let go of it now?"

"Of course, who wouldn't be?"

"Well, some people want to carry on telling the story for the rest of their lives because they get some positive benefit from being thought of as the victim in the accident and they just won't be able to let it go"

"Not me, but what did you mean about 'issues around my neck'?"

The positive benefits of the memory

"Oh yes. The 'me' time you enjoyed when going to the physio. That was your positive benefit for holding on to the injury. It wouldn't have mattered how brilliant the physio was, or what they did. Even though you felt terrific as you left their therapy rooms, your pain would return within a few days, because your subconscious had a positive reason for wanting to continue the treatments."

"Oh god. You mean I stopped myself getting better?"

"In an unconscious way, yes. I'd like you to give a few moment's thought to what those, positive benefits were."

"That's fairly easy. I got out of work early once a week; all the attention was on me for an hour a week; somebody cared about me; I got sympathy from family, friends and work colleagues; it was an excuse I could use not to do heavy lifting, or manual work; oh and it was free!"

"That's quite a list of positive benefits! No wonder your unconscious didn't want to lose them."

"So, how can I help myself get better then? Because I am not likely to get free physio again now."

"You have to find some other ways of achieving the benefits you got. It may be that you do have to pay for a few physio visits, but because you are paying, you'll have an incentive to make the most of the sessions. As for the other benefits you mentioned. Do you really want people just to feel sorry for you?

"Well, no. I'd much rather they liked me for who I am."

"And what about getting some time during the week when you feel the centre of attention?"

"It doesn't have to be every week. There's a massage therapist at the chiropractor's that my wife goes to now and then. I could arrange, maybe a monthly massage."

"And leaving work early?"

"Hmm, not sure about that one. We don't have flexi-time or anything like that, but I guess I could talk to my boss and come to some kind of agreement about working hours that'll allow me to be more flexible if we're not too busy, or if I have worked late on a project."

"And finally, what about the lifting and manual work?

"Well, I don't really do too much of that anyway and I'll just ask someone to help me."

"So, are all those alternatives acceptable to you?"

"Oh yes. They're fine. I just want my neck normal again, so making small compromises like those will be quite easy."

"The one caveat I would give you about this process is not to try and do this on your own. It is a powerful process that requires the assistance of a qualified NLP coach and whilst I can take you through this in probably only a single session, it is not something I'd like you to try and learn."

"O.K., that's fair enough."

Harry resolves his motorway trauma

"What we'll do is tone everything down, change some of the fact to fiction and adjust the ending to a more positive outcome. Ready?" Harry nodded again.

So Mary took him through the process that began to release his trauma over the car crash on the motorway... *{Note to reader – the detail of this process has been deliberately omitted}*.

"Now that you have a new story, tell me what it will be like when you next drive along a motorway, just imagine going along one now, how does it feel?"

"This is great it feels so much better. I am imagining going up the motorway and I can see myself driving really calmly and in control. I am not worried or panicking at all.

Hey! What's happened to the clicking when I look in the mirror? It's gone!"

"Well done. Now that you have a different perception of the trauma, the memory of it will fade away quite quickly, allowing your body to regain its health and release the negative energy of the event.

Traumas can be modified so easily, that we don't have to live with them and let them become more overwhelming than they should be. Some traumas fade with time and this NLP process just gives them a helping hand."

"Could what we have just done be helpful for someone who'd been caught in some kind of terrorist attack, like the 7-7 attack in 2006?"

"Of course. The quicker you can dismantle a trauma and put it behind you the better. If you let the memory of that kind of event run your life, you have given in to the terrorists – they have achieved their goal, to terrorise you.

Now that you have changed your trauma, it won't be something that prays on your mind in old age and becomes overwhelming or a cause of regret.

This change we have worked on today may take a few day's to settle-in as it were, so just give yourself some tender loving care, (tlc) over the next few days, O.K.? Perhaps try a short drive on the motorway after the weekend and build up from there."

"Sure Mary and thank you. I'll see you in a couple of weeks and tell you how I have got on."

"I'll see you on the 26th then. Bye."

Chapter 10:
The Chill-Out Room

Harry arrived at Mary's for his next session absolutely full of himself. He had not only driven on the motorway again, but had taken his family on a trip for the day and driven on three motorways only worrying at the beginning of the day about the fact that he was on a motorway. By the evening and on their way home, he was quite calm about it.

He had erred on the side of caution, sticking to the 70 mph speed limit, but they'd had plenty of time, and they all enjoyed their day out, so it didn't matter that lots of other cars passed them.

He knew Mary would be pleased and proud of him, but the fact that his wife had commented on how brilliantly well he had done was praise beyond any Mary could have given him. He was even rather proud of himself; this was a different experience for him and he wasn't about to go around telling everyone.

As he relayed all this information to Mary, he happened to mention how wound up he had got by the rudeness of other drivers as they tried to get past his car. He couldn't understand it. He was driving at the speed limit and even though he was sticking to the near-side and middle lane, he had been getting flashed and tooted at, as drivers sped right up to his bumper then swerved out to overtake him. It hadn't exactly helped his confidence. In fact, if it hadn't been for his wife telling him that he was doing brilliantly, he might have lost his nerve and pulled off the motorway.

"And how would you describe the feeling of being 'wound up'?"

"Well, sort of like getting more and more angry, but all inside, so my stomach turns in knots and my heart beat gets faster and I start to get really hot and sweaty and there's no outlet for it all."

What is stress

"Oh, I think we have just found our topic for today's session. You have just described some of the most common symptoms of stress. Each person experiences stress in a different way, so something that stresses you, may not affect Jenny or your friends at all. And something that stresses you today, may not tomorrow, perhaps when you have more time to be patient."

"You mean that I get stressed over sitting in traffic, whereas Jenny just thinks of it as an opportunity to listen to the radio or a CD."

"Yes, exactly. Were you aware that, what you call being 'wound up' is how you experience stress?"

"That's stress!? I practically live like that all the time! Especially at work when we have deadlines to meet. Even when I'm not at work I get annoyed with myself, or overwhelmed by something, or obsessed by should's or shouldn'ts, or fret about having a few extra minutes in bed at the weekend. No wonder my friends are always telling me I am too stressed and need to chill-out!"

"And that's exactly the room we need to find in the Manor House to help us do our work this session."

"What? What did I say?"

"The Chill-Out room. That's where you'll learn all about stress and how to recognise your stress and how to overcome it."

"I'll just make a note that what I am feeling are stress symptoms, so I know in the future.

⇒ Symptoms of stress
⇒ Pounding heart
⇒ Sweating or cold and clammy
⇒ Knotted stomach
⇒ Stress is not an event, just my reaction to it
⇒ Something I stress about today, may be fine tomorrow

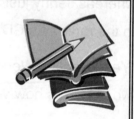

So shall we set our intent and get going then?"

"A most excellent idea Harry. Off you go."

"My intent for today's session is to understand my stress and how to deal with it."

"My intention for today is to help you recognise how you 'do' stress, what the effects might be and how you can best overcome it."

"So, which way is the Chill-Out room then?"

"All I can tell you is that I am pretty sure it is not in any direction you have been so far."

So, Harry walked into the Entrance Hall and turned left towards the East Wing of the house. He walked along corridors of shining wooden floors and thought he must be almost at the end of the wing when he found a double door of highly polished wood with huge brass door knobs. He turned one of the knobs and pushed. As the door opened he saw the most sumptuous room all done in colours ranging from cream to a sort of coffee shade. Thick sound-muffling carpet was underfoot, huge sofas with equally enormous cushions, curtains that promised to keep you snug on a cold wet day and a fireplace stacked ready with logs. There were also floor to ceiling windows in a bay, which let in all the sunshine. The other walls were decorated in a way that Harry couldn't really describe, but they made him feel really comfortable and relaxed. Harry walked over to one of the sofas and sat in the sun enjoying the warmth.

He wasn't sure how long had passed, but the door opened again and Mary walked in and sat in another sofa.

What is stress?

"Well, let's start by finding out what stress actually is. I brought my dictionary from the library, so that we'd have a definitive description.

In the context that we're talking about stress it says this. 'Anxiety burden, hassle, nervous tension, oppression, pressure, strain, trauma and worry'."

"Well, I certainly have a lot of those!"

"Stress is a response to a situation at a particular time."

"Now, let's look at what some of the symptoms of stress are and find out what you are experiencing. An increase in drinking or smoking, frequent headaches, difficulty getting to sleep, lack or loss of concentration, over-eating, jaw clenching, grinding your teeth, waking up in the early morning, back ache, biting your nails (or something similar), being easily irritable, indigestion, mood swings and unexplained muscle aches."

"I could tick a few of those too! Especially the increase in smoking and getting irritable. Oh, and the waking up early and the jaw clenching."

"O.K. At least we know what we're dealing with here. So, let's now find out what your stress triggers are."

Harry made a list. The almost constant traffic queues; the train that's late; the meeting he was going to miss the beginning of; the client who wanted more and more in less and less time; the increase in his mortgage payments, the kids arguing over toys, the junior on the team who always got it wrong, which meant Harry had to put it right. Those were just the ones off the top of his head. He was sure there were more, but he couldn't think what they were.

"I think that's probably quite enough to be getting on with.

"What is your reaction to them?"

"Frustration and irritation mainly."

Have you heard of the fight or flight response?"

"Yes, but I can't really remember the details."

Fight or Flight

"So how about I remind you via a short story. It is the era of cavemen and our ancestor Blog, would go out maybe hunting for berries or plants, however there were also other animals out hunting for food. Imagine Blog meeting a ferocious animal who is licking his lips thinking 'dinner'. Blog's body is programmed with the fight or flight response. But in order to do either the body releases a huge surge of adrenalin and other chemicals into the blood stream. This causes the acceleration of the heartbeat and breathing. It closes down the digestion in the stomach and intestines. The blood vessels in the muscles of the arms and legs dilate to increase blood flow, but elsewhere the blood vessels constrict. Amazing amounts of energy are released so that his arms and legs can move faster, higher or harder than before. Tear and saliva production is stopped and the pupils of the eyes dilate so Blog can see an escape route (or his opponent) more clearly. All this happens so that Blog can live to see another day, rather than being 'dinner' and when it is over and he has outrun the animal, he lies down for a rest before continuing his day.

Now, fast forward from our caveman, to today and let's take a similar scenario in your office.

You are working quietly at your desk and your boss (the fierce animal) approaches and says he needs to see you in his office. You immediately imagine something is badly wrong for him to call you in there, so your fight or flight response jumps into action. Your heart rate increases, your hands get cold, you start to sweat and you suddenly have loads of energy.

Your boss tells you to sit down and you are still expecting the worst but you can't run away and you are not about to fight your boss. Then he says 'I wanted to give you the good news in person. You've been awarded a pay increase and a bonus for all the work you put in on the XYZ account. Without your hard work, we'd never have won the account, nor done such a great job. Well done!'

You are speechless and so shocked that you leave his room with a quiet 'thank you'. However, you've still got all this energy waiting to go somewhere and your heart's still pumping faster than normal. You go back to your desk hoping for a quiet 5 minutes, but someone's waiting to tell you that ABC client is on the phone and has brought next week's meeting forward to tomorrow and they want everything ready by then. So your body goes into fight or flight mode again so that it can cope with the pressure and the amount of work you now have to do before a new deadline.

Do you get the idea?"

"Oh, totally. Blog the caveman only had to use his fight or flight response occasionally and had rest and a normal life in between, but mine's pretty much on the go the whole time, even though I am not actually fighting anyone, nor can I run away – more's the pity sometimes."

The effects of stress

"And what, if any, effect do you think all this stress has on your body?"

"It's going to be pretty bad isn't it? I can tell from the way you asked that question. But I have no idea how bad it is, or how it affects my health."

"Let's think about this together then. I'll give you some suggestions and we'll see what you come up with. How's that?"

"Fair enough, what's first?"

"Think about what I just told you shuts down in your body when it is going through the fight or flight response."

"O.K. You mentioned stomach and guts, so if they are shut down a lot, then it is going to affect how my food is digested. I suppose it could lead to an ulcer in time or maybe something wrong with my guts?"

"That's a good start."

"All this fast heart-beating can't really be good for my heart, so I am guessing there's potential for something to go wrong there.

Oh, if my digestion's not right, that's going to have an affect on whether what I eat is of any benefit to me physically. I suppose it will also have an affect on how long or not, the food stays in my body.

If I am in this response state a lot, then of course I am going to find it hard to sleep and if I don't get enough sleep I know I get really ratty, so my behaviour will change.

"Excellent, you have really got the idea now."

"And if my behaviour changes, that will affect my relationship with everyone I know. So if the kids are being normal kids, I'll just go over the top at them, which means my wife gets all upset at me, which means we don't have a very good evening together."

"The other thing that you may not realise, so I'll tell you, is that prolonged exposure to stress can actually suppress your immune system."

"Which would account for the constant stream of colds, flu and aches and pains I have had in the past."

"To a certain extent, yes. Now, let's find out what you can do about your triggers to help yourself de-stress. Do you have any ideas?"

The de-stress options

"My initial reaction would be to go for a cigarette, but that's not going to help my health, but it does make me breathe deeply. So I could do that without the cigarette."

"That's an excellent idea. Can you breathe in for a count of 7 and out for a count of 1? Why don't you have a quick go at that?"

So Harry did. He counted in his head as he breathed in and out. Doing the exercise now, without any stress made him feel calmer, so he knew it would work for him.

"If I am at work, I could ask other people for help, if I am up against a deadline. I would have to be careful only to do that when I am really up against it, but I am sure it would be O.K. now and then."

"Another great idea. What else?"

"I could go off for a walk in the park that's nearby."

"Yes, and?"

"I could try and just take a break every so often, just get up and walk out to the lifts and back or something."

"That's a great idea. Always move away from where you are working to eat lunch or take a coffee break. It refreshes your mind and allows you to get a different perspective on a problem or issue, or even new ideas.

Far too many people think that they are being heroes or heroines by working non-stop through the day, when in actual fact, taking a break from what they are doing is more beneficial than not taking one. That's also relevant for people who think not taking a holiday will make them look good in the eyes of their boss. It is rarely the case. They are the people who tend to get burnt out and become stuck in their ideas, outlook and ways of doing things. They stop being innovative or useful as team members or individuals."

Harry cringed inwardly at what Mary had said. Whilst he could name at least half a dozen people in his company that worked like that, he too was on the edge of that group.

Mary continued, "This may sound slightly odd, but you could also try standing on a metaphorical or actual chair and looking at the situation from a different angle – literally! It can often help give a totally different and new perspective on a stressful situation, or somewhere you are stuck.

Another thing you might try would be to just stop when you realise you are getting stressed and back track in your mind. Ask yourself what has happened within the last few minutes that caused this reaction.

Once you realise what it is that caused the stress reaction, you can avoid that particular trigger next time."

"I could keep a note of what my stress triggers are in my notebook and if I find myself reacting over and over again, I could ask you for some further help."

"That's a good idea.

I think we have covered stress as a subject, do you feel you know enough to prevent yourself from getting too stressed over issues?"

"I think so. I guess only time will tell. But I will certainly change the way I think about things and how I react to pressure. If I feel myself getting stressed, I can notice what is happening in my body, then start with my breathing exercise and go on from there until it has gone."

"Excellent. That's all you could ask of yourself. And we both know that if something doesn't work, you'll try something different next time."

Harry laughed. "Of course, because it is only feedback!"

Feeling like massive weights had been lifted from his shoulders; Harry left Mary at the door and headed back to his car. Determined that he would be the most chilled-out person on the road!

PART 4

THE LANGUAGE OF WELLNESS

*If your mind can conceive it and
your heart can believe it, then you can
achieve it*

(Rev. Jesse Jackson)

Chapter 11:
The Atrium Of Energy

Mary greeted Harry as he came in for his next session and they sat for a moment in the Entrance Hall, whilst Harry updated her on what life had been like over the last couple of weeks. The last time he had been here, he had worked on how he recognised and dealt with his stress.

He couldn't really explain why, but nothing seemed to be as bad as it had before. Everything seemed somehow, lighter and easier, he even had more energy.

"I'm wondering what you understand by the word 'energy' in relation to your body"

"Well, isn't it what I get from food, so that my muscles work and I can move?"

"That's not exactly what I meant. Let me ask you a different question. Have you heard of any of these words in relation to energy; Chi, Qi, Prana, Universal energy or Auras?"

"I have heard of Chi and Auras, but I don't really know what they are."

"Its how other people and cultures describe the life-force energy that is both within us and surrounds us. The words, Chi, Qi, Prana and Universal energy all describe energy flowing within us, whereas Auras surround us, like a sort of egg-shell.

I'm sure there have been times when you were standing at a function and someone seemed to invade your 'space'. What you experienced then was someone else moving into your energy field.

"Oh yes. I can really understand that! It happens all the time on the tube and I hate it!

"I'm wondering if you would be curious enough to take a look at your energy and find out how it relates to you and your health?"

"I suppose so. I know that sometimes I feel like I have got loads of energy, then there are some people I meet who, no matter how good I am feeling, seem to drain everything out of me and there are days when I just don't seem to have any energy at all.

The whole idea of these sessions with you is to learn about my health and how my mind and body affect it. So, if energy affects my health, I had better find out a bit more about it."

"In that case, let's set our intents and you can get on with your exploration."

"My intent for today's session is to find out what energy is in relation to my body and mind and learn more about how to keep it in balance."

"Excellent. And my intent is to guide and support you in your exploration today."

"So, am I off somewhere in the Manor House then, or am I going outside into the grounds?"

"I think you'll find you can stay here, but it is a sort of outdoors, indoors."

"You know where I am going don't you?"

"Yes. Everyone who finds out about energy does so in this area of the house, so I can guide you there. Just follow me."

They walked for a few minutes by-passing the staircase and the corridors off to the wings, towards the centre of the house, this is where Mary stopped. "Harry, this is the Atrium of Energy. You'll find all you need in here."

Harry looked up at a sheet of opaque glass. "How do I get in?"

'You'll find your entrance as you walk around. I'll wait for you here."

The door marked ENERGY

Harry put his hand out to touch the glass so that he would feel a door. The glass was slightly rough and quite cool to the touch. He slowly started walking to his left, all the time with his hand on the glass.

As he walked, he could feel the glass getting warmer and warmer, then he felt the seam of a door and saw ENERGY etched across the glass. He pushed and almost immediately released the glass door again. As the door opened, there was a cacophony of noise and heat that was overwhelming. Harry wondered if he really had to go into this room. Surely he could just ask Mary

all about it. She seemed to know about most things. He
turned and made his way back to where she was waiting.

"What on earth's the matter? You look white as a sheet."

"I found the door and pushed it open but there was so
much noise and heat that I couldn't face it. Can't you just
tell me all about my energy?"

"Harry, you know it doesn't work like that. Now what
challenged you most about what was behind the door?"

"The heat and noise I suppose and maybe a bit of worry
about what I might find there."

"Let's just stop for a moment. Think about what you just
said to me, the last part of your sentence."

"Worrying about what I might find there?"

"Yes. Where have you come across this kind of thought
before?"

"Oh, the Sound Studio."

"And what did you find out there?"

"That worrying about stuff that hasn't happened is
pointless, because how could I know what might happen

and I am just using old programming and trying to protect myself from harm."

"Well done. So, how could you think about going into the Atrium and what it might hold?"

"As another adventure; knowing that none of the other rooms have hurt me; knowing that I'll learn something about myself; knowing that if I keep an open mind, I'll learn much more."

"Perfect! So, are you ready to go back to the door?"

"Yes. I'll go with the attitude of an explorer; everything I see, hear or meet is a new experience to be savoured and learnt from."

And with that Harry made his way back to the glass door.

He felt exhausted just standing outside the door, listening to the commotion inside. He had to push really hard to open the door, there was so much going on inside the room and things kept banging against the door from the other side.

He pushed his way in and the door slammed behind him, there were little packets everywhere he looked. On the floor, flying around the room, hovering up high, smashing against the walls (that's what he had heard outside); in fact they were all over the place. It was like Christmas gone mad. Hundreds of packets, all wrapped up like presents, being thrown or throwing themselves, around the room. There were also cartoon characters running around, stealing each other's packets and then running off with them.

There were dozens of packets floating around in the air out of reach; they seemed to be held up there as if they were caught up in some wind currents, whilst others hurtled madly across the ceiling. In all the corners there were piles of packets all stuck together that weren't moving.

Harry went to a pile and pulled at the top packet. It eventually came away in his hand and as he turned it, he noticed that on each side was written 'ENERGY'.

Harry pushed his way amongst the crowds of cartoon characters and packets. He found the noise deafening and all this action generated lots of heat, it was a stifling environment. Harry grabbed for the door and fell out into the Entrance Hall, slumped on the floor.

Is that really how my energy is behaving?

Was this really how his energy was behaving in his body? No wonder he often got really tired and had no idea why – he had no idea that this was what was going on. He sat on the floor thinking about what he was noticing about his energy now.

He had had a lifetime of rushing about from one thing to another, giving himself ever increasing targets and challenges to achieve. Was he using all his own energy or was he stealing energy from other people? Or were they stealing it from him? Was that why he got so run down and tired? When he thought about past events, he felt more energised if they were happy, but if they were unhappy, he felt down and flat.

He sat and concentrated on his unconscious and asked himself what percentage of the energy he had in his body was his? A voice came back "about 20%."

He walked back to Mary sitting calmly in an armchair and said "Apparently, I only have 20% of my own energy, where is all the rest?"

Mary immediately congratulated him. "You are obviously getting in touch with what you know in your unconscious but have been ignoring consciously, this is really great and so powerful for you. You are really making progress. What else did you notice?"

"It was a bit like those scenes from *'Charlie and the Chocolate Factory'* I used to read to the children. There were so many things going on, but unlike the book, where there was a lot of order and focus on what needed to be done, in the Atrium it is complete chaos.

There was no order, no balance, no focus, just loads of cartoon characters running riot, stealing little packets marked ENERGY from each other; using so much energy achieving nothing. And there were piles of stuck energy in the corners just not going anywhere, I couldn't even move it."

Harry looked at Mary, recognition dawning on his face, "Oh, this really is my energy isn't it!"

"So, now you have a picture of what is happening to your energy, can you use the metaphor to gain some insights into exactly what you do know about your own energy?"

Harry looked thoughtful yet amused at the same time,
and started explaining what he knew to Mary, whilst
writing in his notebook:

⇒ I have no idea how I am running on
    only 20% of my energy
⇒ When I am in difficult situations, I
    know my energy drops and I feel
    drained for hours. Not sure how that
    relates to the room though.
⇒ I am always very busy in my head –
    plans for this, plans for that, even
    plans for things I have forgotten
    about. So I suppose that is why all
    that energy is flying around the
    ceiling, out of reach.
⇒ When I get overwhelmed with too
    many things to do, I can feel chaos
    breaking out in my head, so I guess
    that's all the cartoon characters
    running around and stealing energy
    off each other.
⇒ People dump on me – they tell me all
    their woes, most of which I can't help
    them with at all, but that seems to
    affect my energy. Is that what all the
    stuck piles are?

"Let's have a look at what you've worked out and what's missing.

Just take a moment and imagine that you have 100% of your energy. How do you think you will feel?"

"Well, great of course."

"O.K., now imagine you have just met someone who wants to tell you all their problems. How do you feel when they have finished talking?"

As Mary said those words, Harry got an immediate image in his head of his friend John.

"I feel as if my batteries have run down. Is this why I am so worn out after speaking with John? He phones and suggests we meet at the pub to catch up. When we meet, he is always fed up and never has anything good to tell me – it is always what's gone wrong in his life! We have a few beers, he tells me all his problems, then he goes off home with a spring in his step and I get home exhausted! Jenny is always saying that meeting John in the pub doesn't seem to be very good for my health, I thought she meant because of the beer!"

"Those sort of people are sometimes called energy vampires and they are normally people for whom 'the glass is always half empty'. They drain you of your energy so that they can recharge their own. By telling you all their problems and woes, they imagine that they have off-loaded all the issues to you and in return you give them time, you listen and you are sympathetic. That to them is energy to live on. There has been an exchange of energy that you were not even aware of."

"Of course - that is where some of my missing energy is! Now I understand the real reason, I could really do with being able to stop John and other people like him, from taking my energy. I don't feel I can stop meeting him, he has been a good friend over the years."

"I'm certainly not suggesting you break off contact with your friends, but you need to learn how to protect yourself from losing your energy to these types of people.

I'd like to take you through how to do that after you've mastered a really simple process for re-energising and clearing blockages. Is that O.K. with you?"

"What do you mean by blockages?"

"Blockages are caused when energy stagnates because it is not moving and gets stuck. The stagnation generally starts after events such as operations or accidents, although it can also be caused by negative emotions building up over time, especially multiple instances of the same emotions.

That's something we'll get onto in a few minutes."

"So, if I could move some of the stagnant energy would that help?"

"To a degree, but there are much easier ways to remedy the situation. Again, I'll get onto those in a moment. Why don't we both go back into the Atrium of Energy and I'll take you through the two procedures I mentioned as well as answering any questions you have along the way."

So they both went back to the door marked Energy and Harry pushed it open. As before, everything looked chaotic, it was hot and the noise was incredible.

"How would you like your energy to be Harry?"

"I'd like all the packets of energy slowed down, there would be none stuck in the corners or high up on the ceiling out of reach and no cartoon characters stealing each other's packets. I would love it if the packets were all just gently circling around and up and down from the ground to the top of the Atrium roof."

"I would like you to really visualise what you have just told me."

Harry shut his eyes tight and imagined his description with all his might. Then he opened his eyes again.

"Let's start with a little more understanding and see where that moves you to. Shall we take a seat?"

Harry turned around to where Mary was looking and noticed two enormous chairs had appeared. He took one and Mary the other.

Mary's explanation

"It's great that you are beginning to understand so much about your energy already. I'd just like to clarify a few things that I am sure you'll find help your understanding and will give you further insights into how energy and health work together.

Different cultures view the human energy field differently, but to start with all you really need to know is that you have an energy flow. You have physical energy, the stuff that makes your muscles work and life-force energy, which is the unseen flow that runs through your body and surrounds it as an aura.

Harry, do you know what the strongest energetic field on earth is?"

"Err, no."

"It's gravity. We know how strong it is, but we can't see it, only the effects of its strength."

"Oh, I never thought of gravity as energy. It is just gravity, but I think I understand what you mean. Just because we can't see or touch something, doesn't mean to say it is not there."

Simply life-force energy

"Yes, that's it exactly. The easiest way for you to understand what life-force energy is like, is to experience it. So, rub your hands briskly together and tell me what you notice."

Harry rubbed the palms of his hands together fast. "Well, first of all, it is getting hotter and there's a sort of tingly friction."

"Good, now slowly move your palms away from each other, what do you notice now?"

Harry concentrated hard on anything that he might feel, "Oh, it is kind of pulling, as if they've got something sticky stuck to each palm."

"Excellent, now try pushing them back together."

"It's like a pressure between them, as if I am pushing against a blown up balloon, or trying to push two magnets together."

"Excellent, excellent. You have just experienced life-force energy at a very simple level.

Grounding is easy

"Right, now that you have an idea about energy, the first of the two procedures that I want to teach you is 'grounding'. Have you heard of it?"

"No, what is it? Is it as easy as what I have just done?"

"For some people, yes. For others, well, they have to try a little harder to achieve it. But it comes easily in time."

"I guess it has got something to do with being in touch with the ground? Like the phrase 'keeping your feet on the ground?"

"You're right about it being to do with the ground. It is a way that we can ensure we are living in the present moment, rather than feeling quite flighty, or disconnected from what's happening around us, or have our heads spinning with all sorts of thoughts and ideas but never actually achieving anything. The phrase you used is great. It is all about keeping one's feet on the ground and moving that chaotic action out of your head and into the calmer waters of your body"

"I can certainly identify with what you said about head spinning but not achieving anything. I spend lots of time doing that. If being grounded will help me stop that and achieve more, then how do I do it?"

"Let me start by repeating that using your imagination in this work is key. It doesn't matter whether you can imagine clearly or not, just pretend you are doing whatever it is we are talking about and that your own spirit, your own inner wisdom knows how to do everything we're about to do."

"O.K."

"The first thing you should do is sit comfortably and quietly with your feet flat on the floor, your arms and legs uncrossed and your back fairly straight."

Harry adjusted his position to reflect what Mary had just told him.

"Now, take four deep breaths and on each out-breath, imagine roots, like a tree, growing out of your feet into the floor and down into the ground. Relax your back and legs into the chair that is supporting you, as your roots reach as deeply as they can towards the centre of the earth."

Harry had an image of some old gnarled roots creeping out from his feet and growing down into the earth, deeper and deeper they went.

"Now just breathe normally and stay connected with the earth through your roots and get an impression of how being grounded feels in your body."

Harry did a scan of his body, like he had done before, and noticed that the pit of his stomach felt quite heavy, so did his feet, and all the things that had been swirling around in his head had disappeared. He definitely felt like he was connected to the earth and it was such a *good* feeling. Not pressured or forced, just comfortable. And he was aware of everything. He wasn't in some dreamy haze. He told Mary what he was feeling.

"This is great Harry, you are doing so well. That is really good for a first attempt. You are obviously one of the people this will come easily to."

"So, all I need to do when my head's spinning is this. I' will get calm and focused and everything will work out?"

"I'm not sure I can make any promises on your behalf, but I can certainly tell you that doing this will make a huge impact on how you work, react, feel and behave."

"Wow, and it is so simple. Why doesn't everyone learn this?"

"If I had my way, they would! I would have it taught in schools! It is such a benefit for everyone! But there I go,

on one of my little hobby horses! Let's get back to you
and your energy.

Clearing, cleaning and re-energising

You might feel stuck energy as a shooting pain, unlike a
muscular pain that is more constant in a given location.
In particular when you have had a traumatic accident,
illness or operation, the flow of your energy is disturbed.
In addition, emotions that we suppress or express in a
negative way can also generate energy blockages.
Some energy can be stuck for years before we realise it
is an issue. We can even take on other people's energy
– such as our parents or friends.

All of your body is connected energetically; every cell in
your body is energy at its core. Even organs that have
been surgically removed, can still be felt energetically.

Keeping your energy balanced and flowing freely is
important, as energy that flows easily keeps the body in a
balanced state of health. Too little energy can be the
precursor for disease or illness, or in the event of too
much energy, you might just cause a domestic fuse to
blow!

You are much more likely to be able to easily fight off any infection or virus before it takes a hold, if your energy is flowing smoothly."

"So no more colds or bugs or flu then?"

"If you were to pick something up, it is less likely that you'll come down with the flu or a cold and even if you did, it would be so much milder than what you've regularly experienced in the past."

"Good, because I don't really want to keep visiting my doctor any more! Nor the chemist!"

"Harry that's great. Just remember what I said at the start of our sessions together and that is written in our contract. What you have learnt and experienced is not a replacement for medical treatment.

So, if you think the time is right to change any medication that you are taking or if you think there is something wrong that needs a diagnosis, you should certainly visit your doctor."

⇒ Energy Vampires (John)
⇒ Grounding!!!
⇒ If my energy is flowing & balanced, I
   will be healthy
⇒ I think my energy is trapped in my
   head
⇒ Unexplained shooting pains = stuck
   energy - it hurts!
⇒ Energy leaves an imprint of a
   removed organ. This is how I can still
   feel like I am getting pain in my
   appendix, even though it was removed
   years ago
⇒ It would be great to get my energy
   flowing well.

Harry had started scribbling in his notebook:

"So, if you are ready, shall we go on to the next procedure?"

"Oh yes, this is where I get to learn how to re-energise isn't it?"

"Yes, so let's start then. What I am about to go through with you was taught to me by Art Giser, who has been working with energy for over 20 years.

Again, the key to this is to allow yourself to imagine it all happening and trust that your spirit or inner wisdom knows what to do.

Let me just explain before I start the process itself. Running your own energy is a very powerful component for promoting health; for clearing your energy field of other people's energies and as a way to transform yourself.

This is just a way of working with your mind, body and spirit. As we go through this process, don't be concerned about what is real or not real. Think about this as being all very metaphorical, play with the metaphors; adjust them if you want to, so that they fit for you. The important thing is not to take them too seriously. When we take them seriously, we try to decide prematurely what is and is not the truth and that only gets in the way. Oh, and if you add in humour, it works even more quickly."

"What, you mean like the cartoons I had in the Atrium?"

"It could be any source of humour, not just cartoons, although they're a good starting point.

I'm going to take you through the process in detail now. Then we'll discuss other ways you can work on your own.

Let's get grounded first, you remember how to do this from earlier on don't you?"

Harry nodded, changing his position.

Mary took a deep breath, and Harry found himself doing the same. Then she began.

"I would like you to imagine on a screen in front of you an image of the earth. It doesn't matter whether you see it clearly, holographically, in 3D, just sort of vaguely see it or even just pretend that you see it. Any of those will work."

Harry sat quietly and imagined himself at a cinema, looking at the earth as if from a spaceship.

"So, see it very clearly, or merely pretend that you see it. Now, imagine the centre of the earth. You can use any image you like, some people get huge crystals, some a molten ball whilst others just see blackness."

Harry went with a molten red bubbling centre. Mary's voice changed tone and depth as he sat there and drifted with what she was saying.

"So just take a couple of easy deep breaths, relax your jaw muscles, relax the point on your forehead between your eyebrows, relax your chest, relax your pelvic area, relax your knees and relax your feet.

Then imagine, or pretend, that the centre of the earth is glowing, sending up beams of light to hit the bottom of your feet and when those beams of light hit the bottom of your feet, they start cleaning the energy centres in your feet and toes, making it easier and easier for the energy to flow into you, whilst enabling you to let go of old emotional patterns, old programming, old limiting beliefs, old mental patterns, old programming, other people's energies.

As the energy cleans and clears your feet and toes, it starts moving up into your ankles, up to your calves, your knees, adjusting all the while to a rate your body is comfortable accepting.

As the energy travels, it cleans and clears your energetic system. The earth energy continues to move up your thighs into your pelvic area, then on up to your diaphragm and a moving ball of that energy gathers at the base of your spine, growing larger and larger so that it fills up the area from the base of your spine to your diaphragm.

(The area around your diaphragm is also known as your solar plexus)

Now, imagine the centre of the earth reaching up with its force of gravity and allow it to grab hold of that ball of energy and to start gently pulling it down to the centre of the earth. As that happens a tube is formed, called your grounding chord, which goes from the base of your spine all the way down to the centre of the earth. Let it be good and wide, wide enough for say a football or a basketball and let the end of it be firmly anchored into the centre of the earth, anchoring and firmly grounding you to the earth.

You should now have a flow of energy, that comes from the centre of the earth, up through your feet, up your legs, into your pelvis and solar plexus (diaphragm area), then turns into a ball and flows back down into the earth through your grounding chord."

Harry nodded. It had been quite easy imagining the centre of the earth and the beam, but he had been

struggling with the concept of the energy travelling
through his body. He had remembered what Mary had
said at the start of the process and just pretended that it
was happening anyway and now, it felt a little strange,
but he thought he had it working.

"Now let's start a second flow of energy. Imagine way
out in space there is some energy that we'll call universal
energy, which is really supportive of you right now. Let it
beam down towards the top of your head. As it
approaches your head, it starts clearing your outer
energy system, which some people call your aura; and let
it clean and clear your energy system until it shines on
the top of your head.

Then it starts cleaning and clearing the energy centres
that are in your head. It starts travelling down the back of
your neck, down your back all the way down to your
pelvis. As it moves through your back it is cleaning and
clearing the energy systems in all the areas of your body
associated with your back.

As this energy goes into the pelvic area, it picks up some
of the earth energy; as it does so, you can play with that
mix, or let your unconscious wisdom control that.

So the universal energy from above, shines on the top of your head and goes down your neck, where some of it breaks off at the level of your throat and travels through your shoulders, clearing and cleaning the energy in your shoulders, your arms, your palms and finally, let that energy shoot out of the tips of your fingers and drop down to the earth.

Whilst the rest of the universal energy continues travelling down your back to your pelvic area, picks up some earth energy and then moves up the front of your body.

As it moves up the front of your body, it cleans and clears the energy centres in the front of your body; through your abdominal cavity, chest, throat, shoulders, arms, hands and back up to your neck and head. Cleaning and clearing as it moves upwards and eventually you let it fountain back out above your head, raining down again to clean and clear your aura.

Any excess energy, or cleaned out energy, goes down your grounding chord and into the centre of the earth.

As these flows are working together, cleaning and
clearing; imagine that your grounding chord has this
wonderful ability to release anything that you are willing
to let go of. Any old emotional patterns, old limiting
beliefs, old mental patterns, old programming, other
people's energies can just flow down through you and
down your grounding chord into the centre of the earth
where it gets reprocessed by the centre of the earth into
positive energy.

Imagine or pretend that all of the energy flows are
happening very naturally, at the same time."

Harry was still sitting in the chair imagining his energy
coming in, cleaning and clearing and going down the
tube to his molten bubbling centre of the earth. He had
no idea how long he had been sitting there, but he
certainly felt deeply relaxed, 'almost asleep' he thought.
He heard Mary talking again.

"Take whatever time is appropriate for you to run this
cleaning and clearing process. You may take 5, 10, or 15
minutes. If you only take 5 minutes a day it will change
your life for the better. If you can afford to take 10 or 15
minutes, that will give you more benefit. The important

thing is to give this process time on a daily basis. That is what will give you the most benefit.

"And lastly, enjoy doing this energy exercise with the understanding that however long you do it for, at the end of it, you will be refreshed, renewed and ready to interact with the world."

Harry was aware that Mary had stopped talking. He didn't really want to open his eyes; he hadn't felt this good in years! He wasn't exactly sure how it had all worked, but he felt truly amazing!

When he did finally open his eyes Mary was sitting opposite him looking at him intently.

"How are you feeling?"

"Pretty amazing"

Harry began to move and fidget in the chair.

"In that case, I suggest you get up and move around, possibly have a stretch and a drink, before we go on to the final section of this session."

Harry came back to his seat and waited expectantly. He couldn't get over how amazing he still felt. Even though he had finished the process over 10 minutes ago now, he still felt great. He was definitely going to do this every day at home!

Protection

Mary continued, "One other process that is relevant for you now will be your ability to protect yourself from those 'energy vampires' we talked about, like your friend John.

There are many different ways of protecting one's energy, but the easiest is to visualise yourself surrounded by a brilliant shell of invisible but semi-permeable white or golden light, a bit like being in a giant see-through egg. Can you do that?"

Harry sat and tried hard to imagine an 'egg' of white light around him but couldn't seem to enclose himself.

"I get to about half way up and then all I can see is a shell broken in half. I can't seem to get a complete egg"

"O.K., let's take it back a stage. Can you visualise a brilliant white or golden egg?"

Harry closed his eyes. "Yes."

"Great, now make your egg bigger and bigger until it is about a foot bigger than you are all over, just nod when you've done that"

Harry nodded

"Now, I'd like you to visualise a small door that will open up to let you walk inside the egg. When you are inside the egg, let me know"

Harry nodded again

"Excellent. Now, whilst you are inside the egg, do whatever you need to, to make it completely see-through."

After a few moments, Harry nodded once more

"You're really doing well here Harry. Just keep that image for a short while. Now, I want you to visualise yourself walking around outside with your invisible shell shielding you, can you do that?"

Harry sat for a moment with his eyes shut, and then he opened them and waited for a few seconds before nodding again. This was hard work, but he was getting the hang of it now. Now he could even keep his eyes open and 'see' his protective egg.

"Excellent work. Now what I'd like you to do is to get up
out of that chair and walk around the room knowing that
your protective egg of light will change shape to allow for
any movement you make, but will still protect you."

Harry got up and started walking around the room, then
he bent down and touched his toes, then he jumped
around, then he stretched up tall, all the time being aware
that he was protected, but not smothered or curtailed in
any way. "This feels really comfortable; do I keep my egg
shell on all the time?"

"That's entirely up to you. What I tend to do is to power
mine up or down depending on what I am doing or who I
am with. So for example, if I know I have an appointment
with people who have drained me in the past, I increase
the power of my protection. If I am on my own, or
perhaps out walking in the forest, I'll drop the protection
right the way down and enjoy whatever energies I come
across.

So, you can change the level of protection to suit your
lifestyle. I'd suggest you experiment with the strength of
your protective shell so that you get to understand what's
right for you in different circumstances."

Harry was amazed. He had had no idea there was any practical solution to people like John. He would certainly put his shell on 'high' next time he went for a drink with him. He was idly wondering what he would need it on at home, with Jenny and the children, or at work with all the hustle and bustle of the office, when Mary broke into his thoughts.

"There are a number of other processes that can help with your energy flows, but some of them will be far more relevant in your later explorations.

For now, trust that the processes you have just gone through and learnt, as well as the one you learnt at the Lake House, will carry out whatever is required in terms of clearing negativity, replenishing you with positive energy and protecting you.

Harry got out his notebook:

⇒ Release
⇒ Re-energise
⇒ Grounding chord
⇒ Earth energy
⇒ Universal energy

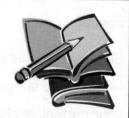

He was sure he had just taken some leaps forward in his understanding of how his energy worked for his health. From now on he promised himself that he would do these procedures at least three times a week. That way his energy would stay as near balanced as he could keep it. He was convinced this would be a change that made the difference to his health.

"I'm so amazed at what I have felt today. It is like I have realised how I can truly help myself. I just promised myself that I would do these processes at least three times a week, and I'll keep my protective shell with me as you suggest, just increasing or decreasing it's permeability. Oh, I can't believe how different I feel."

"I'm really glad you have gained so much insight today. It is wonderful that energy work has resonated with you so easily. I know you'll make the most of what you've learned to help yourself.

There is lots and lots of information on different types of energy and different methods of understanding how to clear or increase it, so I have prepared some notes for you on energy (Appendix 4) that you might want to look into further when you are at home. They will fit into the back of your notebook, sort of like appendices."

"Oh great. Thanks."

Harry flicked through the pages that Mary handed him and saw words like: Shiatsu, TFT, Yoga, Meridians, Ayurveda and Meditation, to name a few; there were many more. Harry made a mental note to look up all the headings on the internet over the next few weeks.

"We have covered a lot today Harry. Is there anything else you would like to ask me?"

"Not at the moment, but I'd like to take a quick look at my energy before we leave here."

"In that case, I'll leave you to it."

Harry stood up and walked over to the centre of the room where he closed his eyes and asked his inner self to show him how his energy was now. He waited a moment and then he opened his eyes slowly. What a difference! The cartoon characters had totally disappeared. The packets of energy that had been flying at great speed around the room high above his head were now hovering around the height of his shoulders. The piles of packets

that had been stuck in the corners of the room had also
disappeared.

Harry looked up towards the roof of the Atrium, high
above his head. He saw a wonderful golden light
beaming down through the glass and reflecting off the
packages that were floating very gently up and down,
hitting the floor as if they were cotton wool and bouncing
up to the roof and again down to the floor. It was a much
more peaceful room than the one he had entered a while
ago.

He gently left the room, closing the door softly.

He found Mary waiting outside for him.

"Well, if that room can change as much as it has after the
work we have done today, then it will be like an oasis of
calm within a week or two!

I'm really going to work on what we have done today. I
just feel so much better now than when I got here."

"In that case, I think we have probably covered quite
enough for this session. Oh, just one extra thing. I'd like
you to keep a diary of all you eat and drink from tomorrow

until we next meet. Take care on the way home; I'll see you again in a couple of weeks."

Harry wondered what the diary was for, but felt so good that he didn't want to lose the feeling. So, with a calm sense of achievement, he made his way home.

Chapter 12:
The Kitchen

Harry met up with Mary after a break of a couple of weeks. He felt in his stomach some slight trepidation about today. Mary had asked him at their last meeting to keep a food diary, so he was guessing they were going to do something about food today.

She had wanted him to record everything he ate or drank, the time he ate or drank it and his mood both before and after eating or drinking.

He had dutifully filled out his diary every day. As he could already see some patterns appearing after only two weeks, he had felt so guilty that he had quietly started adjusting elements of his diet already!

He noticed that he always had a drink and a packet of crisps the minute he walked through the door at home after work; he always had a sugary snack mid-morning and mid-afternoon; he ate far more healthily at the weekend than during the week - that was probably something to do with having more time for eating, or the fact that his wife prepared the food!

Mary greeted him with her normal pleasant manner and asked how he had been.

No matter how much she had been through with him, Harry didn't want to appear nervous about today's session. He put a big smile on his face and said he had been keeping his diary as requested and that he had also been carrying on with the work from their last session. He was already noticing the difference with running his energy and was feeling quite chipper about it all thanks.

"Excellent. Is there anything else you'd like to ask me before we move on with today's session?" Harry shook his head.

"In that case, let's make a start then" said Mary, jumping up from her seat to cross the room.

"Will you pass me your food diary please?"

Harry handed over the document, feeling a mixture of pride at keeping it so well and disgust at some of the things he had actually consumed. Mary scanned it quickly then put it to one side. "Right, let's go to the kitchen then," she said.

Harry stood up to follow Mary. This meant they were going into the Manor House again, but finding the kitchen might be tricky. He had never seen a door marked 'Kitchen' or any kind of area that might represent a kitchen.

Where's the kitchen?

Mary walked across the Entrance Hall with what Harry imagined was an idea of where they were going, only to suddenly stop in front of 4 or 5 unmarked doors and look at him enquiringly. "One of these doors is your kitchen."

Quite flummoxed, Harry stood and looked at the doors. Each one looked exactly the same as the others. On all the other occasions he had been in the house, there had been clues as to the nature of the room, either in the door itself or some kind of label, but here there was nothing.

Turning to Mary he had to admit that he really had no idea which was the right door. Mary smiled her smile, which told Harry immediately that she knew something would happen for him to choose the right door. "Just allow yourself to imagine your favourite meal and you'll know which door to pick."

Oh this was not going to be easy. He thought about all the different food that he liked. Fish and chips, curry, roast dinners, chocolate, Italian, Chinese. How would he ever know?

He told Mary of his dilemma.

"I'd suggest you close your eyes, take a deep breath and allow your unconscious or your imagination to guide you."

He shut his eyes and took a deep breath in through his nose. As he did so, he got the most amazing smell of curry! And it was coming from the far right hand door. He headed straight for that door and pushed it open.

Inside, the room was a hive of activity, with people preparing food on counters, cooking at the stoves or carrying plates of delicious smelling food. As he moved his eyes around the room, Harry could see boxes of fresh vegetables and fruit and he spied not one, but three see-through fridges stacked full of fish, meat and desserts. His mouth started watering as yet another plate of food passed him.

He turned to follow the smell, only to bump into someone carrying a stack of empty plates that all crashed to the floor, making a dreadful noise. The whole kitchen stopped. All eyes were on Harry. He in turn stood frozen to the spot as he looked into the eyes of his old dinner lady from school. He made to help pick up the pieces of smashed plate, but couldn't move. All he could do was swivel his eyes around the kitchen and look at everyone staring back at him. In doing so, he became aware that everyone in the kitchen was someone he had had contact with in relation to food or cooking. From the school dinner lady, to the young man from the sandwich shop that he saw every day, to the waiter at the Indian take-away that he so favoured, to his mother (that was a surprise!), to the kid who worked at the late night kebab and burger bar. All of them were here in the kitchen. No wonder it was so crowded!

Harry stood for a moment wondering what this was all about, then a young woman wearing chef's whites, who he didn't recognise, came over to him.

"Having a bit of bother?"

"Well, yes. I am aware that a lot of the people here are associated with kitchens in one form or another and that I may have crossed paths with them in an eating environment before, but I have really no idea what this all signifies."

"Ah, you are today's guest. Please follow me."

Harry duly fell in behind her and was taken over to a massive table, right in the centre of the kitchen, where he found Mary waiting for him.

As soon as he was out of the main working areas, everyone started getting on with their jobs again and the kitchen once more bustled with activity.

Once sitting out of the way, Harry looked at Mary expectantly, wondering what great gems of wisdom she was about to impart to him. She in turn was looking at him expectantly. Neither said anything for a few minutes.

"Can you wait just a minute? I have forgotten something very important. I'll be back in a second" and with that Harry dashed across the kitchen, this time being careful not to get in anyone's way or bump into anyone, and pushed the swing door, spilling back out into the

Entrance Hall where he ran over to the bench seat where he had left his notebook. He grabbed it and rushed back to the kitchen.

Learning about food

On the table, in front of her was Harry's food diary. "I thought we'd start off with your food diary. Have you had a chance to look back over it?"

"Only last night for a few minutes. We have been really busy at work and it was all I could do to remember to fill it in."

"We have put all the food and drink you have recorded, on that table over there."

Harry looked across the room to where Mary was pointing. It was piled high with take-away cartons, biscuits, chocolate bars, muffins, coffees and sandwiches.

"Oh dear, it looks far worse when you see it like that."

"Let's concentrate on just one day for a few minutes. Would you like to go through your diary for Tuesday of the first week and tell me what you are noticing."

Harry looked at the page and felt his toes curl in embarrassment.

This had been a particularly stressful day at work for everyone and they'd all survived on coffee, snacks, chocolate and burgers, late into the night.

However, when he looked at the feelings and emotions he had written down, most of them said 'frustrated and stressed' before and after, he had eaten. No matter what he had eaten.

"Before we pick another day, I would just like to mention the effect that chocolate can have on a person, other than the sugar high for a few moments."

"Oh dear, this sounds bad too."

"It is not bad as such, just debilitating. Chocolate can drain energy from muscles that are primarily used in movement. So be aware that if you eat too much of it, apart from expecting a sugar slump, you will feel physically tired too.

Now, let's pick another day from your diary. So he looked at Tuesday of last week. The food he had eaten was slightly better that day. But when he looked at his emotions and feelings they again mentioned frustration and stress, as well as boredom this time too. At no point had he put anything like happy, content or satisfied, even after he had eaten.

"I seem to eat when I am frustrated, bored and stressed and by the looks of it, that doesn't change when I have eaten."

"All this stress in your work and life generally, will not help your body digest or assimilate food properly.

It also makes you think you want sugar, salt or fats, when in fact; you are just using those as a cover for how you are truly feeling inside.

Eating at the speed you do and the poor types of food you eat, are blocking the natural way the body tells you that you are full.

You're not giving yourself a chance to taste or savour anything you eat.

Doing the taste test

My concern is that you seem to be eating without tasting, enjoying or even noticing, what you eat or drink. Are you up for taking the taste test?"

"Oh, that sounds fun. Where do we go for that?"

"Just over here at this small table."

They moved to a small table set for one as if in a restaurant.

"The way this works is that you wear a blindfold and I give you dishes to taste and you tell me what you think you are eating."

"O.K. That sounds easy enough."

Harry put on the blindfold and proceeded to taste the dishes that were placed on his table. He wasn't sure what he was eating most of the time and only recognised some very specific tastes like fish and curry. He couldn't actually say exactly what he was eating most of the time.

"That wasn't as easy as I thought it was going to be. How did I do?"

"Well, out of the twenty or so dishes that you tasted, you only got 5 correct."

"Five! Is that all?"

"I'm afraid so. One of the reasons you don't taste flavours will be to do with smoking. It suppresses the efficiency of, or can even kill, the taste buds on your tongue. Smoking also affects your sense of smell, which is a big factor in being able to taste food."

"Oh, I never realised that. I suppose that's another reason for me to give up then."

"It could be, but let's get back to your eating. What has taking the taste test helped you become aware of?"

"That I have no idea what I am eating most of the time. I can only tell what it is because I can see it."

"So what might you do now that you are aware of that fact?"

"I can be more discerning about what I eat. When I eat, I could take more time chewing my food and really tasting it and appreciating it. Oh, and I could stop eating just for the sake of eating. You know, like if everyone is eating biscuits, I could ask myself if I really want it and what benefit it is going to give me, rather than just taking one automatically."

"That's really good Harry. Just by doing what you've mentioned, I am sure you will eat less of what is generally called 'rubbish' food and you will start to make healthier choices about your food too. The fact that you are eating more slowly will allow your stomach to send 'I'm full' signals to your brain, and you won't eat so much anyway."

"I think I'll write those down in my notebook, so I don't forget them, because they were quite good weren't they!"

⇒ Chew and taste
⇒ Ask myself if I really want it
⇒ Eat slowly – is my stomach full?
⇒ Will this food benefit me?

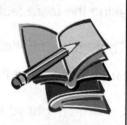

Nutrition and the Nutritionist

"Now that you've done the taste test, what do you know about basic nutrition?"

"That's easy. Nothing! I wouldn't even know where to begin."

"In that case, let's go through a few ground rules with the help of one of our nutritionist friends."

"Mary, what's the difference between a chef and a nutritionist?"

"A chef is a person that has studied for many years in the culinary arts, to learn how to run a successful kitchen. Whereas a nutritionist is a health specialist who devotes their professional activity exclusively to food and nutritional science.

A nutritionist may also advise people on dietary matters relating to health, whereas a chef is more likely to be creative with the food that's available to them."

"Oh, I see. I never realised there was such a difference."

"Harry, I'd like to introduce you to Charlotte, she's a qualified nutritionist and she'll show you some of the basics of nutrition."

Harry followed Charlotte over to another table that was sectioned into colours with different foods in each

section. As Charlotte went through all the different
sections, Harry made notes in his notebook:

Proteins
⇒ Choose low-fat proteins, e.g.:-
  chicken, fish, skimmed milk, low-
  fat cheese, tofu, soya, beans and
  small amounts of nuts
⇒ Eat protein throughout the day, not
  just all in one meal
⇒ Don't eat more than the size of my
  palm
⇒ Make you feel fuller for longer

Minerals
⇒ Major ones needed include: -
  calcium, magnesium, sodium,
  potassium and phosphorus.
⇒ Also some minor ones, known as
  trace minerals, include:- iron, zinc,
  iodine, selenium and copper

Fats
⇒ Four categories – best, good-ish, bad, avoid!
⇒ Best – monounsaturated – e.g. olive, peanut, almond, rapeseed & sunflower oils
⇒ Best fats have a good effect on cholesterol.
⇒ Good-ish – polyunsaturated (cholesterol-free) – most vegetable oils
⇒ Bad fats – saturated – solid at room temp. Mostly derived from meat products (e.g. lard, dripping, butter, cheese.) Beware also of palm and coconut oil!
⇒ Avoid – anything that says hydrogenated in front of it!

Carbohydrates
⇒ Primary source of energy for the
  body
⇒ Carbohydrates contain: - fibre,
  vitamins, minerals and
  antioxidants.
⇒ Good ones found in: - fruit,
  vegetables, legumes (beans), whole
  grains, nuts and low-fat dairy
  produce.
⇒ Bad ones (i.e. highly processed)
  found in:- sweets, biscuits, packet
  snacks, 'instant' foods.
⇒ Eat foods that are not highly
  processed
⇒ Snacks give sugar surges that last
  less than two hours

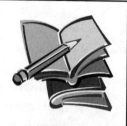

Vitamins
⇒ Vitamin A: fat soluble – found in:-
orange and red vegetables
⇒ Vitamin B (1,2,3,5,6,9,12, also
called different names): water
soluble – found in:-green vegetables,
meats, nuts and whole grains
⇒ Vitamin C: water soluble – found
in:- lots of different vegetables and
fruits
⇒ Vitamin D: fat soluble – found in: -
obtained from exposure to the sun.
also in small quantities from oily
fish
⇒ Vitamin E: fat soluble – found in:-
vegetables, poultry, fish, fortified
breakfast cereals, vegetable oils,
nuts and seeds
⇒ Vitamin K: fat soluble – found in:-
green leafy vegetables and soya

"And as I said, it is the combination of all these different groups that make up a balanced diet."

As Charlotte finished explaining everything, Harry looked at his notes. He hadn't realised there was so much too food!

He could now understand how, for example, eating a heavily meat based dish would put more strain on his digestion than eating say, a vegetable casserole.

He understood why he got a sugar 'rush' and thought he had lots of energy, only to find about 30 minutes later that he was in what he now thought of as 'the big slump', that made him feel tired and lethargic again.

He was now so aware of different types of fats and what each might do to and for his body, especially his heart and arteries, that he was determined to go home and check everything in the cupboards, fridge and freezer! His wife wouldn't be too pleased if he just chucked stuff out, but he could explain to her what he had learnt today and he was sure she would want to change anything that might harm them.

She had been trying for years to lose weight herself, as well as get him to change his diet; mostly via her various fad diets that she went on though! So this would be like she had finally succeeded. He *could* be the new man she wanted! She too could slim down to what she kept referring to as her 'ideal weight'.

If they worked things out, then it would mean the kids would eat better food too. He couldn't stop them if they were out of the house, but by introducing good practice at home, he was sure they would get into good habits that would go with them to their friends and to school.

Harry decided on something then and there. "Charlotte would you help me work out an eating plan that I could take home for myself and my family. So that we can start eating a more balanced diet – at least when we're home."

"I'd be happy to. But before I created anything, I'd like to meet your wife and children. Otherwise, I am rather working in the dark. Here, take my card and call me tomorrow, so that we can arrange a convenient time to meet up. I'll look forward to hearing from you soon. Bye for now."

And with that, Harry finished his notes and made his way back to Mary.

⇒ Eat breakfast like a king, lunch like a prince and dinner like a pauper!

⇒ Vitamin C is highest in any fruit or vegetable that's orange, red or purple

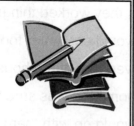

⇒ 'ose' on the end of a word normally means it is a sugar (lactose, dextrose, maltose)

⇒ Eat in the evening before 8.00 p.m.

⇒ Try and eat 2 meat, 2 fish and 3 vegetable meals a week

⇒ Beans don't have to be boring

⇒ Drink plenty of water – at least 1.5l; it helps everything move in, around and out of my body!

"I saw you taking a lot of notes there Harry, I presume you've just learnt a lot that you didn't know, you didn't know?"

"Absolutely! I never knew food was so complicated! Did you know that if we don't have Vitamin C, then we can't absorb iron? And if we don't have iron, we can't make red blood cells. It is all so interconnected, but no one ever really tells the 'layman' about this side of food."

"I'm glad you got on so well with Charlotte." Now, is there anything else we can help you learn in the Kitchen?"

Learning to cook

"I'd love to be able to surprise my wife and cook her a meal that I could be proud of. Do you think one of the chef's might teach me something simple?"

"I'm sure they would, let's go and ask Gerard."

So they both walked over to Gerard, whom Harry presumed was quite high up as far as chefs go, because everyone else in the kitchen was shouting back 'yes chef' or 'certainly chef' to him.

Having heard his request, Gerard asked Harry what he knew about cooking.

"I'll have a go at most things if I can follow a recipe. But most of what I cook is based around mince. You know, like chilli or Bolognese."

"Ah, yes. Student food! What sort of food does your wife like?"

"Erm. Actually I am not quite sure. She always chooses fish when we're out and she's quite partial to Italian food too. Does that help?"

"So, let's do something simple that you'll feel comfortable doing at home. How about a risotto? Then you can make changes to the contents depending on the seasons."

"I thought they were difficult."

"No! They're one of the easiest dishes to make. Come on, I'll show you how and you can make it as I explain it. Then you'll know how to do it at home."

So Harry followed Gerard over to the main kitchen area and learnt how to make a risotto that he could be proud of. By the end of his time with Gerard he felt every bit a 'domestic god'!

"Hey, look Mary! Come and try this and tell me what you think."

"That Harry, is truly delicious! I am sure your wife will love it."

"I'm going to make it for her this Friday. So I don't forget how I have done it here. I just know she'll love it too! Thank you Gerard."

"You are most welcome. Now, if you'll excuse me, I have a kitchen to run."

"I think I am done here now Mary. Shall we leave?"

"Yes, of course."

Once back out in the Entrance Hall, Harry thanked Mary.

"This has been another fantastic session. Mostly because I got to do real cooking, but also because I can help my family change too, by using what I have learnt today. Not just myself."

"I'm glad you've enjoyed it so much. And I am sure your family have already and will continue, to benefit from everything you've learnt over the weeks, but I understand what you mean.

Have a safe journey home Harry. I'll see you again soon."

Chapter 13:
The Orangery

"Hi Mary!"

"Hello Harry; you sound really happy this evening."

"Oh, I am. You remember that risotto recipe I learnt when I was in the Kitchen? Well, I made it for my wife like I said I would and she absolutely loved it! She was also bowled over that I could cook it at all! And Charlotte came to see us and she's given us some guidelines on food choices and ideas about menus. We have all changed a lot of what we used to eat, for food that's far better for us and it is already beginning to pay off! Look!"

And with that, Harry undid his belt to show Mary how loose his trousers were already getting.

"That's amazing Harry. Well done you! And I am sure your whole family is benefiting as much as you are. Just like you wanted."

"It's a bit of a battle with the kids, but we're getting there. Anyway, enough of that. What's in store for today?"

"I was about to ask you the very same question!"

"I feel like I am learning a lot, but there are still some building blocks that I don't have yet."

"And do you know what they are?"

"Well, when I was with Charlotte last time and she was explaining about how all the vitamins and minerals interact with other foods so that the body can use them, she mentioned the immune system.

It was only after I got home and was re-reading all my notes that I realised I don't know anything about it at all. Plus the fact that it also came up when I was in the Chill-Out room.

So, is there somewhere I could go to learn about my immune system?"

"If it is something you wish to learn about Harry, then I am sure there will be a room especially for it. Why don't you go through to the Entrance Hall and I'll follow on in just a moment."

Harry went out to the Entrance Hall and wondered how he would find the room that would teach him about his immune system. He wandered towards the centre of the mansion house, towards the Atrium where he had learnt all about energy, but as he was walking he smelt the strongest smell of oranges. It was as if someone was peeling one right under his nose, but obviously they weren't. He turned away from the Atrium and followed his nose once more. Trusting that, as with the last session, it would lead him to the right place.

He was walking towards the back of the house and the smell was getting stronger as he did so.

He eventually found the source of the smell. It looked like an indoor greenhouse, with lots of small trees in pots lined up in, he noticed, not very straight rows.

He opened the glass door and walked in. The smell was unbelievable but wonderful at the same time.

He sat down under the largest and most beautiful tree and Mary came in and joined him.

"It's a lovely tree isn't it. Do you eat many oranges?"

"Is that what kind of tree it is? I didn't know.

And in answer to your question; not really, although I am sure they will be on our new food list somewhere and I love the smell, does that count?

I do take vitamin C pills every day though. Even before I met Charlotte. Delores in the office told me that she swore by them, she said that all the colds I kept having must mean that my immune system was shot to pieces, so I thought they might be good for me and started taking them every day."

"Have they made any difference?"

"Well I am not sure really, I am not even sure how I would know. I still get colds, but they don't seem to last quite so long, so maybe they have helped."

"Shall we set our intents before we become too involved in today's subject and this wonderful perfume?"

"Mmm. It is lovely isn't it? My intent is to find out about how my immune system works for and with, me."

"My intent is to guide you to the resources that will help you support your immune system."

Harry's immune system

"So, when you think about your immune system, what picture is conjured up in your mind?"

"A hard metal military tank, that's broken down, going rusty, bits missing and holes in the sides, basically, shot to pieces and useless."

"Was that image ever any different?"

"Oh yes. It used to be a black tank, really strong armour, had guns blasting and killed off whatever or whoever the enemy was."

"So you really have taken on Delores' view of your immune system."

"I suppose so."

"Do you recall in the Ballroom of Beliefs how you can take on other people's views of the world, which are really not yours at all?"

"Yes. Oh, that's what I have done with my immune system isn't it. That never occurred to me when I was in the Ballroom."

"Never mind, you had a lot going on during that session. At least you are aware of it now.

Can I suggest you go over there and meet old Bayleaf
the Gardener; see if he can give you a different
perspective on illness."

So Harry took himself over to where old Bayleaf was
pottering amongst the trees.

"Hello young fella. Come to see my trees have you?"

"Well, actually, I was wondering what happens when one
of them gets ill?"

"Funny you should say that. I have been very worried
about this tree. You see, this is the sunny side of the
Orangery and I had a few days off last week. When I
came in this morning, she was looking a bit sad.

It was really hot last week and although I left strict
instructions about watering, I think she may have run a bit
short."

"Oh, I see. So what will you do?"

"Firstly, I have to make sure the environment is right for
all my trees to flourish. Water is first on the list. Without
the right amount of water, none of us can flourish! It's not
just for trees. This will certainly help her to find her own
strength to recover, but I don't think that is all.

You see the earth in this bed? It's looking very powdery; I think it would do her good to have a little natural feed. Being indoors, the trees can't get as much natural nutrition from the ground as they would like, their roots don't go down deep enough and they can wilt quickly when something is not right."

"And what do you mean by natural feed?"

"Oh, I only use organic feed. Manure, worm farm wee, home created compost and the like. I do as much to promote her natural healing as I can.

I'm not one of those gardeners who try to force their trees to produce copious numbers of oranges by using chemicals. I just want them to remain as healthy as possible.

"What would chemicals do then?"

"Well lad, they create a false sense of security, so the tree doesn't think it has to do any of the work. The more chemicals you give it, the weaker it becomes and the more susceptible to any infections.

It's a bit like you or I taking pills for everything and expecting to be cured each time. After a while, you have to take stronger and stronger pills to get the same effect. If you had just helped your body create it's own defences, it would be able to fight off most every infection quite easily.

This tree has been great at overcoming any form of disease in the past. She just needed the right support from me, to help her own defences along."

"That sounds pretty impressive."

"That's nature for you. If you give it a helping hand now and again, it knows how to cure whatever is wrong.

You can't force nature. Have you ever thought of how a little seed knows how to blossom into a lovely tree that can bear fruit? Us gardeners can't control that. All we can do is to give the trees the best opportunity and the space they need to develop.

If we have to prune a tree to prevent it becoming too big, or cut off a lower branch, or there is an accident and it loses some bark, the tree will heal itself by sealing the wound with more bark, we are not instructing it how to do that, the tree has learnt for itself. But if we cut a tree when it is weak it is unlikely it will ever recover. Its natural healing is so weak; it just can't make the extra effort.

The trees are the experts on how to grow branches, make shoots, what to do in which season etc., not me. I just try to provide the best environment and support for them to flourish. I also like to give them a hug of encouragement sometimes – I think it makes a difference!"

Harry thanked Bayleaf and left him to his ministrations for the tree and returned to sit with Mary.

"I'd just like to make a couple of notes before we go on."

⇒ We know how to heal ourselves if we have the right support
⇒ When we don't heal there is something else wrong
⇒ Water
⇒ Nourishment
⇒ Love and encouragement
⇒ Protection

"Now Harry, can you remember what we discussed in the Sound Studio about how you speak to yourself?

This idea of Delores's that your immune system is all 'shot to pieces'. How do you think your immune system feels about that?"

"Ghastly! I feel quite sick just thinking about a part of me that is all shot to pieces."

"Such is the power of your internal dialogue and the pictures you show yourself."

"I want to change this right now. It is horrible. It doesn't convey anything about how I want my immune system to be."

"So how do you want your immune system to be?"

Harry brought out his notebook. "Let's see, it needs to...,"

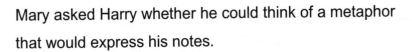

⇒ Learn new things every day
⇒ Access all information at any time
⇒ Be able to change its mind when it finds a mistake
⇒ Be very clever
⇒ Know which are my cells
⇒ Identify & eliminate intruders
⇒ Be strong
⇒ Adapt to changing environments and conditions

Mary asked Harry whether he could think of a metaphor that would express his notes.

"Not really any one thing. What I get is a cross between a robot, my original tank and myself."

"Could you make something up that would fit? Remember, it doesn't have to be real."

"In that case, I have invented a robot tank that has human intelligence programmed into it, so it knows the difference between friend and foe. It can shrink to the size of a single cell, or grow to the size of a chieftain tank. It also has an exponential memory chip, so it can remember new things and recall everything it has ever learnt."

"That sounds perfect."

"Yes, I think it is! So, how do I go about replacing the old shot up tank with this wonderful new one?"

"As you so rightly said a moment ago, your immune system changes and learns every day. It learns things and puts them into immediate action to safeguard you. So all you need to do, is direct its learning just a little bit per day, to help you move towards your goal of this fantastic, new, adaptable and powerful tank.

Take a few seconds to remember what you have learnt already in some of the different rooms, because I am sure you already have some ideas about how you can do this."

"I could start with creating a picture of what the final tank will look, sound and feel like."

"Good. And what else could you do?"

"Oh, I can keep telling myself in an affirmation how knowledgeable, flexible and responsive my immune system is."

"Excellent. Anything else?"

"I could change my static final picture into a movie that starts with the original shot to pieces tank and rebuilds it into the new super tank."

"Oh well done Harry. That is perfect! Remember to start your movie every day, from the latest re-build. Never go back to the original start point. Then, if you run your updated daily movie faster and faster until it becomes a blur, it will get into your unconscious even faster and your results will appear more quickly."

"Oh, I didn't know that bit. I will just make a note of that if you don't mind.

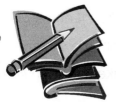

⇒ Run my movies faster and faster until they become a blur. The info will get into my unconscious and get results more quickly.

Successes and mistakes

Mary reminded Harry about their discussion on positive intent they had had in the Study.

"Now that you are already working on improving your immune system, what do you think might be the positive intent of all the minor illnesses you have had? What has your body been trying to tell you about your immune system?

"That it wasn't working?"

"Do you think that accurately reflects what was going on?"

"No, not really. If it hadn't worked at all, I would be in a hospital. I think it was struggling to work properly."

"And have you any ideas why it was struggling?"

"No, not really."

"O.K. Let me give you some ideas about how your immune system can become compromised, then you can take over with some ideas of your own.

Not taking care of yourself; not getting enough quality sleep; strained or poor relationships. Now, do you think some of that relate to you?"

"Stress has got to be in there somewhere, because that's what I have had lots of! And possibly something to do with my diet?"

"Those are two that are very specific to you, but also affect many other people too. Good. Can you think of any others?"

"I suppose if someone was taking drugs it would have quite an effect on their immune system. Do tea, coffee, alcohol and cigarettes count as drugs? Would pollution have an impact too?"

"All excellent ideas Harry. There is one other big area that can affect the immune system. Think of emotions and how you used to think and talk."

"Oh, of course, negativity!"

"Brilliant! Anyone who is continually negative will, in time, affect their immune system. Have you ever noticed how happier people always seem to be healthy? That is no coincidence!"

"But what about when as children or teenagers we are given jabs? How does that work?"

"Vaccinations are just very mild doses of an antigen that triggers an attack response from the immune system, so that it learns how to deal with that particular microbe, in advance. It is preventative, rather than waiting for a person to contract the full blown disease and having to go through a possibly painful or dangerous healing process. The immunity is learnt."

"So, what happens with auto-immune diseases then? How does the immune system go wrong?"

"I, along with many scientists and researchers, wish I could answer that, but you have sort of answered your own question. The immune system somehow gets confused and starts to attack its own body's cells as if they were intruders."

"Is that what happens with cancer too?"

"No. That is different again. Everyone has cancer cells in their body now and again. However, most peoples' immune system can identify them and remove them.

In very simple terms, a cancer cell is just a cell that has mis-formed and loses all the programming of a normal cell about replication, life-span and death. It is as if the

immune system has dropped a stitch in its knitting and
one of the cancer cells gets away to eventually form a
tumour.

Whilst we are on this subject, I might as well tell you
about allergies too.

When someone develops an allergy, their immune
system has got the wrong information stored and over-
reacts to whatever the allergen is. So, in hay fever for
example, instead of ignoring the pollen as something that
is totally harmless to the body, the immune system starts
a full attack on the pollen."

"Heavens, I never realised that's what happened. So it's
just a bit of information that has been stored incorrectly in
my immune system that causes the sneezing, itching,
bunged up nose and rashes?"

"Yes. Amazing isn't it? You can of course, easily and
quickly re-programme your immune system, so that it
realises things like pollen are not harmful and learns a
more appropriate response. It is one of those NLP
processes that only takes a short while but has an
incredible effect."

"Maybe we could do that before the next hay fever season starts? Right now, I would like to concentrate on getting my immune system back to my new super-dooper image of it."

"Of course. Let's back-track slightly. Now that you are aware of what can affect your immune system in a negative way, how could you help re-build it?"

"Well, won't it be most of what is negative, but in reverse? So, all the positive things. Like good relationships, good diet, being happy, staying calm, taking time to relax, living in a clean environment and of course, having fun and being positive!"

"You have it exactly! And how many of those things you've just mentioned will you be doing?"

"Well, I will try to do all of them. I'm not sure that I can change my environment at work much, but I can certainly do so at home. That's another reason to stop smoking and I'm sure if I did, my immune system would benefit.

You know, now I come to think of it. I don't really want to smoke any more. Over the weeks, I have found so many reasons for giving up and I know I'll be so much more healthy if I do. As well as the fact that I can save almost £30 per week! That would be enough to pay for a lovely holiday for all of us by this time next year. You know what Mary. I am going to give up! From right now!

"Oh, how excellent! That really will help your health; in all sorts of ways."

A bit of fun to help it along

I would like you to leave with something that is a little bit of fun, to help you on your way to that amazing immune system you are heading for.

I was taught this little rhyme by Suzi Smith, one of my trainers and it has stuck with me ever since. In fact I often hum it whilst out walking the dogs. I'll teach it to you, it is really easy to pick up.

It's to the tune of 'Short'nin' bread', which I'm told is an old American folk song, I think from the slave era, but I call it the 'Happy cell song'."

Mary started humming the tune of Short'nin' bread and tapping her foot in time with the music.

"These are the new words that have replaced the original lyrics. They are specifically for health." And Mary sang

"*Every little cell in my body is happy,*

Every little cell in my body is well.

Every little cell in my body is happy,

Every little cell in my body is well.

I can tell, every little cell,

In my body is happy and well.

I can tell, every little cell,

In my body is happy and well.

That's it. Very simple, but very effective."

"It is a bit like an affirmation, only you are singing it."

"I never thought of it like that before, but you are right. It is a sung affirmation. Shall we have a go at singing it together?"

So that is what they did. After a couple of verses it became infectious and Mary and Harry could be seen jumping around the Orangey, laughing and singing, feeling more and more healthy by the minute.

As Harry left Mary's house he already felt that his immune system was on the way to a full recovery. He had a spring in his step as he walked to the beat of the 'Happy cell song', that was still repeating through his head and he felt really great about his decision to give up smoking. Just wait until he told Jenny!

Chapter 14:
The Bedroom

Harry bounced into Mary's practice room, a big grin on his face.

"This is different!"

"Yes, I know. It's the new me!"

"So tell me what has changed then. I am really curious to know what you have been doing."

"Well, after our last session, I went home and had a long talk with Jenny. It was long overdue and we sorted out a lot of what has been worrying us. During our conversation, we realised that we have both been worrying about the same things, but never told each other, in case it caused a row!

I ceremoniously burnt my last packet of cigarettes and I haven't had one since. I haven't even craved one, which I have to admit I am quite surprised at. In fact, just the smell makes me feel slightly sick.

Jenny and I have really gone full throttle with the eating plan that Charlotte gave us and if the kids don't like it, we encourage them to at least try it, but they don't get anything else instead.

All of us have started to lose weight! I have had to buy some new trousers and Jenny is thrilled at the weight she is losing because she's not really trying and she says that she isn't obsessed with food like she used to be on her various diets.

The kids seem to have calmed down too. Both at school and at home. I'd just like to get them away from watching TV or playing on the computer, but that's another issue. Oh and one of the best things is, that I've been going to bed and sleeping through the night, without tossing and turning for ages worrying about things or, waking up at silly times of the night. The only thing is, I am not sure what I have done that has brought about this change."

"Wow Harry! That is amazing! It is so great to hear you say all this and to see how much you have changed in your posture and demeanour. You have certainly come a long way from the person who originally walked in on that first day.

I get the impression from what you said about your sleep, that you might like to find out what you have done, so that you can use the resources and strategies, or at least know what they are, for the future. Is that correct?"

"Yes, is that possible? I know that all the other times I have explored the Manor House, it has been because I have a problem, but I would really like to know what I did to change my sleep."

"Of course it is possible. Have you any idea where you would find the information you are looking for?"

"I thought probably the Bedroom would be the place to explore. I'm guessing that it will be on one of the upper floors of the Manor House, above the Drawing Room or the Ballroom of Beliefs."

"In that case, I shall let you make your way up there and I'll be up shortly."

Harry left Mary and walked through the Entrance Hall and up the central staircase. He followed the stairs up to the second floor and stopped at the top. He shut his eyes and asked himself 'should I go right or left? His reply was the very faintest snoring coming from down the landing to his left. So he headed in that direction.

As he approached what seemed to be the only door on the landing, the snoring got louder and louder. He turned the large brass handle and opened the door.

Meeting himself asleep

Asleep on the bed he saw; no, it couldn't be. He looked again, rubbed his eyes then looked again. There was no getting away from it; he was looking at someone who was the spitting image of himself!

Harry walked over to the bed. He couldn't quite believe what he was seeing, but remembered where he was. Instead of learning how to change though, this time he wanted to know what he had done to change without realising it. He had not however, expected to meet himself!

He wondered when the sleeping him would wake up. He looked so serene and untroubled in sleep. Was that a smile on his lips too? Harry wasn't aware people smiled in their sleep and wondered if that was how he looked now too.

He moved a chair closer to the bed and sat down and very quietly he whispered "are you awake?"

There was no response from the sleeping him, so Harry said slightly louder "I said, are you awake?"

With a start the him in bed harrumphed and still with his eyes tight shut muttered

"Well, I was in the middle of the most amazing dream, until you just woke me up!"

"Oh, I am sorry. But, you are me aren't you?"

"In a manner of speaking, yes. And your reason for waking me is?"

"Well actually, to ask you how we, because I am assuming that you sleep as well as I now do, sleep so well."

"How we sleep so well? But if I am you, then surely you must know?"

"Actually, I don't. I have only recently realised that I am sleeping through the night and not waking up worrying and I really have no idea what I have done that has caused the change. And I *would* like to know, so that I can keep a note in my notebook and learn what I did, so that I can use the strategy or resources elsewhere in my life."

"Oh, I see. So where do we start this then? Perhaps if I tell you what we had already learned, but didn't realise we were using, that might be a good place."

"Yes, that sounds like a good idea. I'll just get my notebook ready in case there is anything I want to jot down."

Now, let me see. I think we started to sleep slightly better after we had visited the Library."

"Really? That long ago?"

"Well, that is where we learnt to set our intent, and if you remember, we started setting an intent to sleep through the night, just before we got into bed."

"Oh, yes. I never really expected it to work though and I am sure I still woke up a lot."

"Yes, we did. But what we didn't notice was that the period of time between getting into bed and falling asleep got ever so slightly shorter each week and that the period of time between falling asleep and waking up worrying got ever so slightly longer each week."

"It did? I'll certainly make a note of that then. What else?"

> ⇒ Setting intent *really* does work - very subtly!

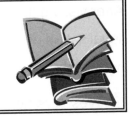

"Then when we had visited the Sound Studio, where we learnt about the self-talk that we hear in our head. We got a tip from Mary that week, but I'm not sure whether we wrote it down or not. Check back and see if we made a note about writing down all the things that we go over in our head before we try and sleep."

Harry flicked back through his notebook to his visit to the Sound Studio and sure enough, there was the note.

"Yes, I had made a note, look. And I have been doing that. The writing everything down I mean."

"And it has obviously helped, because we no longer wake up worrying about missing or forgetting something, because we know we have written it down."

"O.K., so that's another strategy. What else have I done that I can't remember?"

"After visiting the drawing room, we created a visualisation of sleeping peacefully through the night every night."

"Oh, yes. I remember doing that for about a week or so, then I forgot to do it any more. I can't remember the last time I ran that visualisation."

"Well, that has worked too! Honestly, we really must start trusting our unconscious more! We are running all these new strategies and getting brilliant results, but we are forgetting to give ourselves or our unconscious any credit or praise for achieving the results we wanted. Maybe we should write that down in the notebook!"

So Harry did. Not just because his other-self had told him to, but because he really thought that giving himself and his unconscious praise would help things along enormously, (which it did).

⇒ Give myself and my
  unconscious praise!

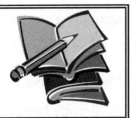

"This is amazing. I really didn't think that each time I came to the mansion, I would learn something that would help me sleep. Is that all, or is there more?"

"Oh much more! Are you ready?"

"Sure, fire away!"

"Do you remember our visit to the Ballroom of Beliefs?"

"Yes, that was quite a hard session, but I don't remember anything about sleep in that session."

"Well, there wasn't anything that we worked on specifically, but just by recognising that we had a belief about not being able to sleep, we started the process of changing that belief in our unconscious."

"So you mean that I wasn't even aware that I was changing, but I was changing anyway?"

"Yes! Fascinating isn't it?!"

"Actually, it's a bit mind blowing. I'm not sure I can get my head around that concept."

"Well, right now that doesn't matter. What matters is that it is already happening. Our unconscious is way ahead of our conscious mind and did it for us! Think of it this way. We filled the washing machine and set the programme then walked away. The machine did the rest and we let it get on with it, knowing that it would do a good job."

"Oh, that's easier to follow. I think I might make another note about that.

⇒ My unconscious can work without
   my conscious input.
⇒ Just give it the details or even just
   an idea and trust that it will
   finish the job correctly

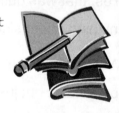

You know, I can't believe how much I have learnt that has affected my sleep. I really thought I would still be struggling, but just listening to you, it seems that almost every time I came here, I learnt something that helped. Even if I wasn't aware of it."

"So, where do you think we learnt our next piece of information that helped us?"

"I suppose from the Lake House of letting go. But I am not sure how that helped me."

"Learning how to release all that old baggage has really helped us to let go of the silly day to day niggles that used to keep us awake."

"So, now we have the hang of this, let's just run through the rest of the rooms we have been in and pick out what we think we have learnt in each that has helped us with our sleeping."

"The Chill-Out room"

"That one is easy. The breathing exercise that I learnt. I think I'll put that together with the Lake House as a note because they sort of go together.

⇒ Let go of daily baggage
⇒ Breathing relaxation
⇒ Ground myself every day

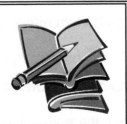

"The Atrium?"

"Oh definitely grounding! Actually, that could go in with the notes I made just now."

"What about the kitchen?"

"Hmm. I'm not sure if that room had any affect on my sleep. Have you got any ideas on that?"

"Why don't we write this down in our notebook, ready?"

⇒ If I am not going to be able to eat before 8.00 p.m.; have a lunch instead!
⇒ Dinner like a pauper
⇒ Spread out my intake of food across the whole day, not all at dinner!
⇒ Stay off the caffeine and cheese after 6.00 p.m.

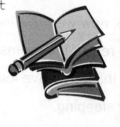

"Do you think the Orangery had any affect?"

"We think it is more likely that our newly enjoyed sleep has had an effect on our immune system."

"That would be right. It fits in much more with what I learnt in the Orangery."

"So, there we have it. All the things we have learnt over the weeks that have affected our sleep without us even realising we were doing anything differently. And we get all the benefits of proper sleep now too! We really struck gold with this room!

Now, if we can be excused. There is a dream we would dearly love to get back to!"

And with that Harry's other-self snuggled back down under the covers, shut his eyes and drifted back to his dream.

Harry crept back over to the door and quietly let himself out. He had a lot of information, but was that really all he needed to know?

He found Mary sitting outside on a small sofa on the landing.

"I thought you would have come into the room with me."

"I did peek in to make sure you were O.K., but you and your other-self seemed to be making such good headway that I didn't think you needed me at that point. So, I came back out here and waited for you."

"Well, I have lots of notes and I now realise how much I have learnt over the time I have been coming to see you, but I am still not sure if I have missed anything. I mean, I still don't really know what happens when I sleep."

"Would you like me to elaborate a little?"

"Yes please, if you can."

The good things about sleep

"During sleep your body increases the rate at which it creates and mends cells.

Full pattern sleep (that's getting through all 5 stages of sleep) helps support your immune system, rejuvenates your nervous system and relaxes your muscular and skeletal systems.

It is a little known fact that people who regularly have unbroken sleep for between 5-8 hours live longer than those who sleep less than 4, or more than 9 hours, or are subject to broken sleep patterns."

Harry didn't know any of that, but he made a note of it in his notebook.

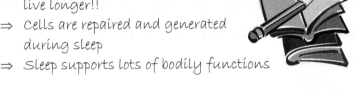

⇒ 5-8 hours of regular sleep helps you live longer!!
⇒ Cells are repaired and generated during sleep
⇒ Sleep supports lots of bodily functions

What a lack of sleep causes

"So, having told you what sleep can do, let's look at what a lack of it can cause."

"Well, I think I could probably tell you that!"

"Go ahead then, let's make a verbal list."

> I get really irritable with all sorts of things, not just people.
>
> I can't work properly
>
> I lose interest in conversations
>
> I feel dizzy
>
> I eat lots of sugary things and drink lots of coffee to try and keep awake

"Well, that's a good start, but they are all things you notice. Do you know what a lack of sleep can do to your body?"

"Oh, no, not really."

"Some of the things you mentioned obviously, but also, nausea – which you may actually have felt in the past, which is why you would reach for a sugary snack.

Decreased immune system function – which could explain your almost constant stream of ills in the past.

An increase in blood pressure and water retention), which might have been the cause of your bloated feelings and reddish tone.

A slowed reaction time – that one's rather dangerous if you are driving.
Oh and the big one; you age faster!"

Harry made more notes…

Not enough sleep can cause
⇒ Irritability
⇒ Lack of concentration
⇒ Nausea
⇒ Decreased immune system function
⇒ Increase in blood pressure
⇒ Water retention
⇒ Slow reactions
⇒ Faster aging!

Just a few extras

"Wow! I would never have thought of those. Is there anything else that I should make a note of that will help me?"

"You might wish to add these to your notebook."

And as Mary spoke, Harry wrote.

> ⇒ Create and stick to a sleep ritual
> ⇒ Sleep regular hours – even at weekends
> ⇒ Remove the TV from the bedroom

"They all seem quite simple and easy to accomplish.

This has been a great session, everything seems to be coming together and I now understand how everything inter-relates.

It's not just sorting out my eating or me stopping smoking. It's learning about and doing everything else as well. That is what gives the roundness to this whole process."

"I am very glad to hear it. Do you have any other questions about sleep before we leave the mansion house?"

"No, but I was wondering if there was anything left for me to find out here."

"I think perhaps one last learning might be appropriate. Especially as you mentioned earlier wanting to get your children away from the TV and their computer games.

We can take a look at that in 10 days, if you want. Goodbye Harry."

Chapter 15
The Adventure Play-Grounds

"Hello Harry. As this is your last session with me at the Manor House and as the sun is out and it is such a lovely warm day, I thought it would be pleasant walking in the grounds. Shall we?"

"Oh yes. I haven't really taken much notice of anything outside the house. Well, apart from the route to the Lake House that is."

Taking a walk

"So, tell me. How have you been since your visit to the Bedroom?"

"Really great! All the thing's I have learnt are falling into place and I am using them without even thinking about them. Well, most of them at least.

My session in the Bedroom has confirmed to me that everything is intrinsically linked in one way or another and that I can't just view my body or mind as separate components of myself. Whatever my mind thinks, my body will react to and whatever I do to my body will have a knock on effect in my mind and hence my body again."

"Those are quite significant insights for someone who a few weeks ago just took a pill for anything that was wrong."

"I really have changed Mary. Even people I don't know very well are telling me how great I look these days. I dread to think what they used to see!"

"Let's not worry about what they used to see and concentrate on what they now see."

"Yes, I know. Sometimes I wonder if they really mean me when they are saying things like that, but they look straight at me, so it must be me!"

"Of course it is you!"

"I still find it amazing. I just wish I could get the rest of the family to do everything that I have done and feel such benefit from it."

"Remember, that this has been your very personal journey, it will not be the same for other members of your family and friends. Also timing is all important. This sounds to have been really great timing for you, when you were determined to find a better way. The timing always has to be right for the individual when they are open to change.

Perhaps you could start in a very simple way with your children. Do you remember at the end of our last session, you mentioned your kids and how you would like them to do something other than watch TV or play computer games?"

"Yes. I haven't made much headway there unfortunately."

A lack of exercise

"Well, I was wondering what *you* do when you get home in the evening? Or what hobbies you have, or what sports you play."

"Oh dear. When I get home, I sit in front of the TV!! Somewhat hypocritical isn't it?"

"That is one way of expressing it. Is there anything that you would like to do but for some reason haven't up until now?"

"I used to love cycling. Before Jenny had the kids, I used to belong to a local cycling club. Nothing very official, just a group of us who used to meet up at weekends and one weekday evening during the summer months and go off cycling somewhere. There is a big forest near where one chap lives and we would often cycle through there. It was great fun. We used to have a laugh, a bit of gentle competition to see who could go the fastest or do the biggest jump, or get across the deepest stream and we would end the evening with a pint in the local pub. Then at weekends we often went out for a half day ride in the countryside.

All that stopped as soon as our son was born. There just never seemed to be time to go out. I sometimes see cyclists and wish I was still doing it myself."

"Well could you? Now that the children are that much older?"

"I'm not sure how Jenny would take to me being out for half a day each weekend, or even one evening a week. Then there is all the ferrying around we have to do with the children, to this party or that friend's house."

"So tell me. What do you think you could do that wouldn't impact family life?"

"It would have to be something that I could do during work hours, or on the way to or from work, but without encroaching too much into my evening."

"Do you mean something like go to the gym?"

"Heavens no! I hate the idea of gyms. I can't bear to pay someone for the privilege of using some static equipment, whilst surrounded by TV screens and blaring music!"

"Let's do a brain storm, of all the things you could possibly do as we walk and talk."

"Brain storm?"

"Yes, it's a term I use when all I am doing with someone is throwing out ideas. It doesn't matter how absurd the idea is, or how unrelated to the topic. If an idea pops into your head, you say it."

"Oh, I see what you mean. We call that, having a power-thought session, in our office."

Ideas outside the gym

"That seems a much nicer way of saying it. O.K. then, let's do some power thinking as we walk."

"Well, walking."

"A great idea. It's free, you can do it anywhere and it will all go towards your 10,000 steps per day."

"What do you mean 10,000 steps per day?"

"That is the recommended minimum number of steps a person should take per day. I believe the number has been suggested by health experts across the world."

"How do I know if I am walking that many steps?"

"You get yourself a pedometer. The one I have is quite simple and just clips to my waistband, see."

"So you walk 10,000 steps a day?"

"Actually, I walk more than that most days, but I try and ensure I do at least 10,000."

"I wonder how many I've walked so far today."

"Try standing over here. This will tell you."

"It's just a tree stump, how is that going to tell me how many steps I have walked today?"

"Trust it."

So Harry stepped on the tree stump and was amazed when a deep voice said "3,067."

"That's all? Are you sure?"

"3,067"

Harry got off the tree stump and looked at Mary who was smiling.

"I'm not even going to ask how! I'll just make a note to buy one of those pedometers like you have."

⇒ Buy a pedometer
⇒ Do at least 10,000 steps per day

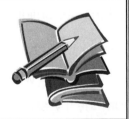

"If you look on the internet when you get home, you will find lots of sites that give suggested walking plans or programmes to help you get fitter using your pedometer.

So, now that we have covered walking, what other exercise would you consider doing?"

"I would like to get back on my bike. Maybe I could cycle to and from the station instead of having Jenny drive me and pick me up each day. That would work. So long as it wasn't raining."

"It is certainly better than sitting in a car every day. At least you are making some effort. Do your children have bikes?"

"Oh yes, but they only seem to use them in the summer with their friends in the park."

"If you can't go out with your old cycling group, how about taking your children out through the forest?"

"I never thought of that. There are some places we could all ride. Even when it's wet. That would get them away from the TV and computer and Jenny could have some time to herself!

I wonder if any of the lads I used to ride with have kids now. Maybe we could all go out together."

"So that would be a wonderful all-round solution."

"I think it's one that will certainly happen. I will just write that down, so that there is no chance I can forget it!"

⇒ Take the kids riding through the forest each week
⇒ Jenny gets time for herself
⇒ Get in touch with the lads from the cycling club – do any of them have kids too?

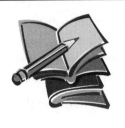

"Now, let's think about when you are at work. What could you do there?"

"Not a lot. I tend to spend most of my day sitting on a chair. Although I do have to go up and down between our floors a lot to see one art director or another. I could use the stairs instead of the lift. It's only a couple of floors, but 'every little helps' as they say."

"If it's only a couple of floors, you could start of walking up them and eventually perhaps, run up them!"

"Let me just add that in to my notes.

⇒ Take the stairs at work
⇒ Start off walking up and
   down them
⇒ Graduate to running up and
   down them

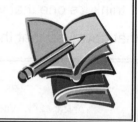

I am going to be so fit, and all without the aid of an expensive gym!"

As they had been walking they had passed various small clearings in the woods, but Mary hadn't mentioned them, so Harry had kept quiet. At this clearing however, he could see rope ladders reaching up into the trees and his curiosity got the better of him.

"Mary, what are all these clearings for? And where does that rope ladder go?"

"The clearings? Oh, they are all workout areas for the adventure course that is hidden within the woods here. The ladder you noticed goes up to the tree-top walk-way."

"Oh, that sounds fun! Have you ever done the course?"

"Not me, but lots of my clients have done it in the past. They all seemed to enjoy it tremendously. Would you like a go?"

"Oh yes!"

"In that case, I'll call through to one of the adventure instructors and ask him to meet us at the start of the course."

They carried on with their walk, enjoying the tranquillity of the woods and throwing out ideas of what Harry could do to exercise without going to a gym or having to run, until they came to a big clearing far away from the house

Waiting there was a giant of a man dressed in a combination of army combat and high-tech sports gear. He smiled and waved as Mary approached.

"I have another guest for you Jim. Harry would like to do the adventure course, can you take him please?"

"Surely. Pleased to meet you Harry."

Harry took Jim's proffered hand and as he shook it wondered if he was choosing the right thing. Jim's handshake was what one might call solid. He didn't look like he was made of muscle, but in Harry's eyes, he looked super fit.

Oh well, too late now. Besides, it had looked like fun and it was probably the only opportunity he would have to do something like this.

Harry walked off after Jim.

First there was a short chat about safety, then some information about how to do the course, what to look for, how to judge distances high up or across water, and finally, Harry was kitted out with all that he might need to complete the course.

"Am I doing this completely on my own?"

"No, I'll be behind you to keep an eye on you, but I won't interfere, unless you really need my help."

So, taking a deep breath, Harry started the course.

At first it seemed really awkward. There was lots of uneven ground and he couldn't get into any kind of rhythm as he half ran, half walked. He would lose his stride climbing the rope ladders, but get it back as he followed the well worn track through the woods.

He decided to stop trying to think about what and how he was doing and just let his body move towards, over or under whatever came next. This was a much better strategy, for in doing so, he found his natural stride and the course became much easier to follow.

He even had time on the tree-top walk-way to admire the view all around. Across the woods towards the house and from there over the meadow towards the lake. It really was beautiful.

He got back onto the track through the woods and started noticing things he would never have normally seen. Trees, bird song, rabbit markings, stream beds, animal tracks through the fallen debris of the woodland floor.

He found himself climbing ropes and A-frames, crossing streams on fallen logs, scrambling over mounds of earth and rope, even climbing a small rock face.

And he loved it! The more he did, the more he enjoyed it, and the happier he felt. When he eventually got to the end of the course, he was ready to do it again, he just felt *so* good!

The exercise high

"Oh Mary, that was absolutely fantastic! Brilliant! Amazing!

I feel like I've just conquered Everest or landed on the moon or something equally amazing!"

"That will be all the endorphins rushing around your body."

"What are they?"

"They are a chemical that is released by the body under certain circumstances, one of which is participation in over 30 minutes of aerobic activity. That is, exercise that works the cardio-vascular system. They are sometimes known as the runners 'high'. Amongst other things, they generate a state of mood enhancement which is what you are feeling now."

"I just had a brilliant time and it was great fun! Was that all endorphins?"

"No, they are just the after effect. You really did genuinely have a good time, all on your own!

And doing something you really enjoy or, is important to you, generates more energy. And the opposite is also true; doing things you hate or are boring drains your energy."

A family affair

"I'm sure my son would love something like this. Do you think they have kids' versions?"

"I'm sure there are some somewhere. I think it would be a case of checking the internet for somewhere local that you could go. Perhaps you could do it together."

"Oh yes, that would be fun. A real father and son outing! I'll just make myself a few notes."

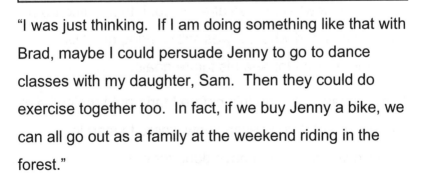

⇒ Find an adventure course for Brad and me to go around
⇒ Endorphins – the body's natural 'high'
⇒ Aerobic exercise for over 30 minutes releases endorphins
⇒ Doing things that are important to me generates energy

"I was just thinking. If I am doing something like that with Brad, maybe I could persuade Jenny to go to dance classes with my daughter, Sam. Then they could do exercise together too. In fact, if we buy Jenny a bike, we can all go out as a family at the weekend riding in the forest."

"You are certainly sounding very enthusiastic about exercise now Harry."

"Well, if I can include my family, we will all get the benefits of being healthier; we will be doing things as a family, or at least child and parent; and the more we do, the more I am sure we will want to do. It's the final piece of the jigsaw for my own health and I can share it with my family. It's a total win, win!

Let me just make sure I have all the notes about what we have spoken of today. Yup, I think I have everything."

Saying goodbye

"In that case Harry, let's walk back to the Entrance Hall."

On the way back to the mansion house, Mary and Harry talked about how Harry had changed and what he had learnt. About what he had already put into practice from his learnings and what he was still working on. His achievements so far and his future goals.

"I know I have told you this before Mary, but I really am a changed man! I don't even know where to start in thanking you for all you have done for me."

"I think you will find that you did pretty much all of it for yourself. I was just around with a helping hand. You have come a long way and learnt a lot of lessons Harry. Be proud of yourself!"

"Do you know one of the things I'm looking forward to most?"

"I have no idea."

"Going back to the chemist with all the old bottles of pills and potions that I got prescribed, for him to dispose of. I can't wait to see his face! And I also plan to encourage my friends, when the time is right for them"

"In that case Harry, I will bid you farewell and wish you all the health and well-being you desire for your future. Remember, there is always more to learn, stay curious and you will enjoy your future journeys too."

"Thank you Mary, you have made such a difference to my life. Good bye."

Appendix 1
Harry's Contract With Mary

I, Harry Winthrop am committed to creating a coaching alliance with Mary Hibbert that will support me as I clarify and realise my goals and move steadily toward achieving the health and well-being I want to have. Mary agrees to hold all content of our sessions confidential, to the extent permissible by law.

I want to work with Mary to shape the health coaching relationship to best meet my needs by:

Learning about my own motivation.

Helping me get in touch with my own body and its wisdom

Noticing my values and what is important to me.

Co-designing strategies that will support me.

Refining and changing a strategy or behaviour when it doesn't fit for me.

Helping me to develop and retain curiosity for things that happen to me.

I give Mary permission to:

> Challenge me with powerful questions.
>
> Request that I take action.
>
> Hold me accountable for actions that I commit to.

I understand that health coaching is not a substitute for proper medical consultation for physical, mental and psychological illnesses. It is not intended to replace the services of a qualified medical practitioner. It is provided as complementary to other avenues you may be pursuing.

Appendix 2
Mary's Tips On Visualisation

Visualisation is the use of your imagination. It is an ability we all have. You can use the power of your imagination to create what you want in your life.

The more you use this power creatively, the easier you will find you gain the benefits, as your mind helps your body to process your unconscious requests.

Starting the process

Just close your eyes for a moment and imagine a cat meowing for its food.

Did you get a picture? Or just a sense that the cat was there? Or could you hear the cat perfectly?

Let's try another example.

What does the word 'clambering' bring to mind? I get a picture of clambering over rocks at the seaside. What did you get?

Now, think of something you did recently that you enjoyed. Really get a sense of being back in that time &

place; notice the colours and shapes that were around you; hear the sounds that surrounded you, feel the sensations that you experienced. As you run the memory through your mind, really be part of the memory, seeing it through your own eyes, not just an onlooker to it.

Excellent! You have all it takes to be able to visualise successfully!

If you think something's missing - don't worry!

Lots of people when they first start to visualise can't 'see' a picture when they close their eyes. Some worry that 'nothing seems to be happening'. For some people, as they focus on say their wedding day, the picture 'develops' in front of their eyes, just like the film from an instant camera, and as they turn their attention to different aspects of the day, more pictures develop.

Visualisation is not only about being able to see pictures.

We will go through some simple exercises to help you achieve successful visualisation.

A simple exercise

Read through the rest of this exercise and then close
your eyes and try it. (We have used a room, person or
animal as an example all the way through. You can use
whatever you wish)

Step 1 - Relax!

Sit or lie comfortably and take 4 deep breaths. Try and
breathe all the way down into your belly.

Breathe in for 4 seconds, hold the breath for 2 seconds
and breathe out for 6 seconds.

Step 2 – remember something familiar

Close your eyes and remember something very familiar
to you. It could be a room or a person or an animal.

Remember as much as you can about what the room,
person or animal look like; any colour; shades of
darkness or light; shadows; brightness; depth of colour.

Step 3 – remember sounds

Still with your eyes closed, remember any sounds that
you associate with the room, person or animal. What
pitch are they; how loud or soft; is it constant noise,

silence or intermittent sound; is it sound you appreciate and enjoy or not; can you make the sound yourself?

Step 4 - remember physical attributes

Keep your eyes closed and recall physical sensations associated with the room, person or animal. Any smells associated with your choice; hard or soft surfaces; textures; density; height; feel.

Step 5 – using your imagination

Now, imagine that you are somewhere you would love to be right now. It can be somewhere you have been before, or just a place that you make up.

Wherever it is, think of all the details that you would like to be there. Be as precise about the place as you can be.

Result – how you visualise

Whatever process(es) you used to imagine the scene you just chose in your mind, is how you naturally visualise.

Make a note of how you did it, for future reference.

Visualisation works best if you know exactly what you want. You can repeat the visualisation often and you can give it lots of energy.

Whilst it is admirable to want to visualise world peace, if you are just starting out on visualisation, it is recommended that you start with small and easy ideas or goals.

This will allow you to maximise your success and build on your visualisation skills day by day.

If you wish, write down your visualisation and get someone close to you to read it out to you. Alternatively, record your own voice on an mp3 and play the recording back to yourself. Or, you might ask your mentor, coach or support group to talk you through your visualisation.

What to do next

However you decide to work, setting the goal of your visualisation is your first task.

Make sure that you have a very clear picture, feeling or sound (or preferably all three!) of the end result, exactly as you want it to be.

Whatever you decide on should be in the present tense (i.e. it already exists); with yourself fully associated in the situation (i.e. you are involved with it, seeing it through your own eyes, seeing your own hands and feet, not looking in on it).

The art of visualisation is to think about it both frequently and clearly. Not just if you are meditating or having some quiet time, but to think about it throughout your day, in a calm relaxed way. It is important not to put too much emphasis or force into achieving the result.

Whenever you think about your visualisation, try to get the sense that you **really do** have the power to bring this about. Think about achieving it, in a positive, calm, joyful way. Imagine yourself being in the result of your goal. It will also help if you make positive affirmations (see the Sound Studio chapter in the book) about the result of your visualisation.

Continue to visualise your goal until you have (a) achieved it or, (b) it is no longer relevant.

Sometimes what we think is our goal (and therefore becomes our visualisation) changes to something different as we ourselves change, grow and develop.

N.B.

Please be aware that visualisations should always be for the positive benefit and for the higher good of anyone concerned. Anything negative that is visualised will certainly come back on you, faster than you could imagine. This is the basic law of karma ("what goes around, comes around" "as you sow, so shall you reap").

Appendix 3
The Lake House Releasing Process - In Full

From the work of Art Giser

Get grounded first

Sit comfortably and quietly with your feet flat on the floor, arms and legs uncrossed and your back fairly straight. Take 2 or 3 deep breaths, allowing all your muscles to relax, especially your jaw, chest, abdomen and feet.

Each time you breathe in, breathe all the way down into your belly and as you breathe out, feel all the muscles in your body relaxing.

Set up your grounding chord so that it is on 'release'.

The process

Close your eyes and imagine a deep sea, or lake, or river out there in front of you. Give it whatever surroundings you like.

Imagine that at the very deepest point in this water is a magnet. This magnet is so powerful that it can attract negative beliefs, old negative programming, old emotions, limiting beliefs that no longer fit you, or other people's energy out of the cells in your body.

Put your attention on the magnet and imagine that it is gently and powerfully pulling anything negative out of your cells. Trust that your unconscious mind will only get rid of whatever is not of benefit to you, or is not serving you. Your unconscious is very conservative so if it is willing to let go, you can trust that it will not let go of anything you need.

Whilst the magnet is working, don't bother to try and analyse what is coming away. You may get images, or feelings, or you may hear sounds as the negativity leaves you. Whatever your experience is, this is right for you.

Allow the magnet to pull out whatever form this negativity takes and suck it into the water where it can dissolve and drift down into the centre of the earth for processing back into positive energy.

Other people's energy may not dissolve, just let that sink
to the sea/lake/river bed and let it go back to wherever it
originated from.

If you don't feel like anything's happening, just imagine
that you are removing whatever is blocking the negativity
leaving you.

If it still seems blocked, imagine removing whatever is
blocking the block.

If you are still not getting a sense of this working, imagine
removing the block, that's blocking the block, that's
blocking the block!

At this point, there will be nothing left to block anything.
Now, let the magnet do its work.

Just imagine the magnet working for as long as you feel
is appropriate.

When the magnet has finished its work, dispose of your
image and magnet. Some people like to explode it into
millions of tiny pieces that fly out into space; some people
send it down into the centre of the earth where it is
reprocessed into positive energy; some people wrap it up

and throw it in a metaphoric bin. Do whatever works for you.

When you have disposed of your image, imagine a golden ball of positive healing energy is hovering above you. Pay attention to the ball and imagine it growing and sparkling with positive healing energy.

Now, allow the golden energy to filter through your skin and fill any gaps that have been left in any part of your body since the removal of the negative energy. Let any excess just go into your grounding chord.

When to run the process

This process is recommended to be run at least twice a day (on waking and prior to going to bed). It can be run at any time if you wish to remove any negativity that you may have picked up in a particular circumstance.

It was right for you

Whatever you experienced is right for you at this time. Please do not compare yourself with anyone else when running this process. There is no definitive 'correct' way that things should happen.

Appendix 4
Energy – Mary's Notes For Harry

Meridians

In traditional
Chinese
Medicine, it is
believed that the
body has lots of
interconnected
channels running
through it called
meridians
(Chinese: jing-luo
经络), that carry
'life force',
'spiritual energy'
or 'vital energy';
all similar names
that mean the
same thing, and

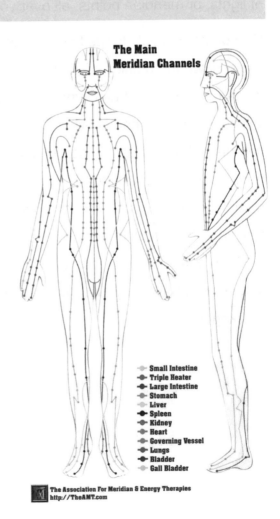

**The Main
Meridian Channels**

- Small Intestine
- Triple Heater
- Large Intestine
- Stomach
- Liver
- Spleen
- Kidney
- Heart
- Governing Vessel
- Lungs
- Bladder
- Gall Bladder

The Association For Meridian & Energy Therapies
http://TheAMT.com

also sometimes known as 'chi' or 'qi'. Along each channel there are various points.

Think of your energy being distributed all over your body like fairy lights on a Christmas tree. You have hundreds of lights, or meridian points, all over your body.

One of the easiest strings to locate, is by running your finger down the outside of your leg, just where the seam of your trousers is. Follow the line of the seam and you will have run your hand over around 20 points along a meridian. If you press along the seam gently you may notice pain at intervals that can indicate blocked meridians. Now just like the annoying habit of Christmas tree lights, if one point goes off then it is probable the next few will go off too. To get your energy flowing well, you need to have all your little lights on, with no blockages.

Chakras

In Hinduism and some other Asian cultures, a chakra (Sanskrit: cakra चक्र "wheel") is believed to be a connection to, or of, energy residing in the body.

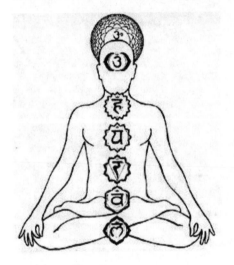

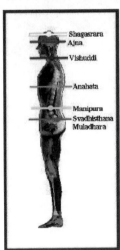

Chakra	Colour	Primary Functions	Associated Element	Symbol
Crown (just above the head): sahasrāra,	white or violet; may assume colour of dominant chakra	connection to the divine	space / thought	
Third eye (centre of forehead): ājñā,	indigo	intuition, extra-sensory perception	time / light	
Throat: viśuddha,	azure blue	speech, self-expression	life / sound	
Heart/Lung: anāhata	green	devotion, love, compassion, healing	air	

Solar plexus (over diaphragm): manipūra	yellow	mental functioning, power, control, freedom to be oneself, career	fire	
Sacrum: svādhisthāna	orange	emotion, sexual energy, creativity	water	
Root: mūlādhāra	red or coral red (shown)	instinct, survival, security	earth	

Think of chakras as either wheels or circles that are aligned in an ascending column from the base of your spine, to the top of your head and extend out past your physical body. They are believed to vitalise and be associated with the inter-actions of mind, body and spirit. The function of the chakras is to spin and draw in universal life force energy, also known as prana, to keep the spiritual, mental, emotional and physical health of the body in balance.

Other energy resources

There are many others styles or types of energy, of no lesser importance, but I can only give you a sketchy outline of what they're about. I suggest if you are interested in finding out more, you explore the internet for further information.

Shiatsu massage - there are many different styles, although the basic premise is 'diagnosis and therapy combined'. One style will be what you might consider deep massage techniques, whilst another focuses on gentle pressure to unblock energy that's become stuck.

Ki Therapy and Acupuncture – these two therapies work in a similar way, using pressure and needles respectively, on various meridian points to change your energy flow, in order to restore balance within the body, mind and spirit.

Reiki - is a form of energy healing developed in Japan. Practitioners use a technique similar to what's known as the 'laying on of hands' where they act as channels for 'ki' energy which is guided through their hands to heal a person wherever they may need healing.

Emotional Freedom Technique (EFT) - a modified form of the original Thought Field Therapy (TFT). Both techniques use a specific order of tapping to help release negative emotion that has been stored within the body, causing energy blocks and therefore imbalance within the body.

Physical techniques - Chi-Kung, sometimes written as Qi-Gong, and Tai-Chi teach a person how to move their own energy, clear blockages and maintain health. You will be able to find local classes for these too. In fact, all martial arts have both a spiritual and energetic aspect to them; it is just that we tend to hear about the physical practice and its effects.

Glossary Of Words

Affirmation: A positively worded phrase set in the present tense, which is repeated frequently on a daily basis. Ideally 33 times per day for 33 days for optimum effect/benefit.

Allergy: The physiological equivalent of a phobia, a rapid or repeated overreaction to a specific stimulus on the part of the immune system. An allergy is an inappropriate reaction to something that is not life threatening in itself.

Antigens: It is identified by the immune system at something that is foreign and should be attacked.

Autopilot: When you have become so competent at a skill, you no longer need to think about it consciously.

Aura: The energetic field that surrounds each living thing. Often described as 'egg shaped' and frequently said to be different colours depending on the state of health.

Baggage: Slang for physical or emotional events that are remembered and possibly referred to, but of no significant use or benefit to one. "Stuff that's past it's sell by date."

Beliefs: What you take as true. The generalisations one makes about ones reality.

Chunking: Viewing an idea in big chunk (big picture), or drilling down into more and more detail (small chunk). A way of making a large task more manageable by breaking it down into small chunks.

Confusion: A state you are in when you are struggling to achieve what you want. It is a natural feeling when learning something new (conscious incompetence).

Conscious: Anything you are currently aware of. The top of the iceberg, your unconscious holds the rest of the information of the iceberg.

Endorphins: A hormone released in the brain, which has a calming effect on the body and makes many people feel good. Endorphins can be generated by exercise and even conscious focus.

Energy: (Universal) Often used to refer to a higher entity that has no religious affiliation. A source of energy that can help with replenishment of personal energy or can provide healing energy. **(Life)** In eastern medicines; the energy that is believed to run through and assist in balance of, the body.

Framing: When you change the frame around a picture, let's say from brown to red, the picture can take on a different look or feel as other colours are highlighted. Framing is the way you label your experiences to give them meaning. Simply by changing the frame (re-framing) you can change the meaning of your experience and remember things very differently.

Generalisation: A process whereby one experience comes to represent a whole group of experiences.

Grounded/Grounding: Being in a state of connection and awareness within the present moment.

Immune System: The immune system is a collection of cells that identifies and kills non-host cells.

Intent: One's wish for the highest benefit for those involved in an activity or task.

Internal dialogue: The conversations you have with yourself to resolve a problem to help you think things through.

Introjected voices: Those voices that are heard inside one's head, but that originate from someone else, e.g. a parent or teacher. Often 'heard' in phrases that start with 'you'. e.g. "you should know better."

Mind's eye: The mental picture you paint of an object or word that you can see by recalling that image from your memory.

Nutritionist: A Nutritionist looks not just at what you eat, but how your body absorbs, processes and utilises the nutrients you receive through the foods you choose to eat on a daily basis.

Overwhelm: A feeling of not being able to cope with too many diverse stimuli. You can't understand 'how to' get out of your confusion and achieve what you want, typically by continuing with the same thought patterns.

Phobia: An irrational sense of fear when confronted with a common object, activity or situation. A very common form of anxiety.

Positive Benefit: The hidden benefit of a seemingly negative behaviour.

Programming: The way you do things, as a result of experiences you have had

Re-framing: Changing your way of understanding a statement or behaviour to give it another meaning; changing the frame. The ability to reframe allows you to make meanings of events, which have previously been difficult or impossible, in ways that work for you and create desirable emotional states.

Resources: Anything you notice or need that will assist you to hold or regain a state.

Self-talk: The chatter and conversations that go on in our heads.

State: Simply, how you are at any given time.

Strategy: The way you do something and the process you use time and again for doing it – some work well, but others do not.

Trauma: Any event that has had a profound affect on one. Often remembered with full visual, sound and feeling associations. Can be the trigger for onset of disease, as the immune system is temporarily compromised immediately after the trauma.

Triggers: Whatever triggers a habit or strategy.

Unconscious: Everything that is not in your current awareness. This is the part of the brain that runs 'in the background', being responsible for recording all the events in your life and running parasympathetic body functions (e.g. breathing, heart beating), etc. The events of your life affect how you see the world etc (some people call this your subconscious).

Visualisation/picturing/imagining: The process of capturing, holding and recalling a mental image or photograph.

Contacting The Authors And Other NLP Practitioners

You can contact the authors of this book through their web-sites or via e-mail.

Olive Hickmott	www.empoweringhealth.com olive@empoweringhealth.com
Sarah Knighton	www.breakingboundaries.co.uk info@breakingboundaries.co.uk

Workshops and seminars based on the content of this book are run on a regular basis by Olive and Sarah. They are focused on changing and improving one's health and have no pre-requisite learning.

For more details about either the workshops or seminars, please see the web-site of the book.

www.youtoocandohealth.com

Other NLP practitioners are available throughout the world. We recommend that you go to a recognised training establishment and find out if they hold a list of qualified practitioners whom they are willing to recommend.

New Perspectives

New Perspectives has brought together a unique set of books, especially for those who wish to explore how they can be more the person they want to be. The objective is to offer you, the capability to start your own personal development journey around the specific area that you are currently focused on, such as:

⇒ Improving your general health
⇒ Recovery from illness
⇒ Overcoming learning difficulties
⇒ Moving on from a long standing health problem
⇒ Wanting to feel you are doing a better job of being a parent, son or daughter
⇒ Building your confidence
⇒ Reducing stress and letting go of what is no longer important
⇒ Improving family and business relationships
⇒ Better communications with yourself and others
⇒ Coping with a recent promotion or career change
⇒ Setting your goals and stepping up to the challenge
⇒ Losing anger.

Each book is focused on specific issues you may wish to address. If you find a particular book of value to an immediate need in your life you may become curious to understand more about other aspects. We would encourage you to move on to other areas that you may feel appropriate.

The books are written by co-contributors, who are experts in this field or have first-hand experience of the material or topic being addressed. Some authors are NLP Master Practitioners, with many years of experience of different aspects of personal development and professional coaching. The collaboration between the authors is crucial to the success of what they have achieved, and could not be done individually – an inspirational collaboration.

The books include many stories, metaphors, examples, client experiences, pictures, dialogue and sometime workbook pages to fully illustrate the point and help the reader move forward. They will be challenging, as personal change can only be achieved if people are prepared to be open to how they can to achieve what they want.

As individuals grow within themselves they find that:

⇒ Some of the day to day worries of modern living melt away
⇒ Their focus on the things that are really important is increased
⇒ A calmer and more grounded individual appears, less effected by any negative personal experiences, more able to cope with whatever life presents
⇒ Illnesses change and start to shift
⇒ Energy and fun increase – often more than they ever thought possible
⇒ Your inner wisdom shines through.

Index